Trauma
Culture, Meaning and Philosophy

Dedication

This book is dedicated to my mother, Peg Bracken. Her wisdom has always been an inspiration.

Trauma
Culture, Meaning and Philosophy

PATRICK J. BRACKEN PhD, MD, MRCPsych

University of Bradford

W
WHURR PUBLISHERS
LONDON AND PHILADELPHIA

© 2002 Whurr Publishers Ltd

First published 2002 by Whurr Publishers Ltd
19b Compton Terrace, London N1 2UN, England
325 Chestnut Street, Philadelphia PA 19106, USA

Reprinted 2003

British Library Cataloguing in Publication Data
A catalogue record for this book is available from the
British Library.

ISBN 1 86156 280 2

Contents

Foreword   vii
Acknowledgements   xi

Chapter 1   1

Introduction

SECTION I   TRAUMA, MEANING AND PSYCHIATRY   15

Chapter 2   17

Enlightenment, psychiatry and the nature of mind

Chapter 3   45

Post-traumatic anxiety

Chapter 4   63

The limitations of cognitive approaches to meaning and trauma

SECTION II   A PHENOMENOLOGICAL APPROACH TO MEANING AND ITS LOSS   83

Chapter 5   85

Heidegger's account of human reality

Chapter 6   112

A Heideggerian approach to psychology and psychotherapy

Chapter 7   **130**

Meaning, anxiety and ontology

Chapter 8   **151**

Authenticity in question

SECTION III   MEANING AND THE CULTURE OF POSTMODERNITY   **165**

Chapter 9   **167**

Modernity, postmodernity and the question of meaning

Chapter 10   **189**

Responding to postmodernity

Chapter 11   **204**

Conclusion

Endnotes   **228**
References   **236**
Index   **249**

Foreword

Trauma: Culture, Meaning and Philosophy, Pat Bracken's remarkable synthesis of practical innovation with deep philosophical insights, illustrates, paradigmatically, why the 1990s, although rightly proclaimed as 'the decade of the brain' in psychiatry, turned out also to be the decade of philosophy. Hand-in-hand with dramatic advances in such areas as brain imaging and the genetics of behaviour, the 1990s witnessed the Philosophy Group in the Royal College of Psychiatrists growing to become the College's second largest section (with 1600 members), a wide variety of other groups springing up around the world, a number of international conferences, several new Masters and PhD programmes, new research, and a new international journal: *PPP – Philosophy, Psychiatry, and Psychology.*

Bracken has been at the cutting edge of these developments. Armed with doctorates in both philosophy and psychiatry, he has drawn deeply on the continental philosophy tradition in his clinical practice. In particular, he has sought to engage with the thought of the French philosopher, Michel Foucault. With others he has established an inner-city home treatment service for people with severe mental illness that is based on an explicit philosophy of care rather than on the theories and techniques of traditional psychiatry. In this he has worked to establish new models of user–provider partnership in the organization and delivery of services.

In *Trauma: Culture, Meaning and Philosophy*, Bracken extends this double-barrelled philosophy-plus-practice approach to the work of the German philosopher, Martin Heidegger. At first glance there might seem to be little connection between the arcane phenomenology of a politically dubious mid-twentieth-century academic (Heidegger was an active member of the Nazi party for a short period) and the practical exigencies of clinical work in psychiatry at the start of the twenty-first century.

Bracken's philosophical insights, however, stem directly from his personal experiences working with victims of violence in Africa in the aftermath of civil war in Uganda. Severe trauma destroys the meaningfulness of a person's world. Western paradigms of trauma management, as Bracken describes in Section I of this book, aim to restore meanings by therapies that focus on the intrapsychic worlds of individual people. But Bracken and his co-workers found this paradigm increasingly unsatisfactory. For the meaningfulness of the worlds of those with whom they were working turned out to be primarily interpersonal rather than intrapsychic, and social rather than individual.

Enter Heidegger, then. For Heidegger's great achievement was to re-orientate phenomenology from the intrapsychic focus of its founder, the German philosopher Edmund Husserl, to the interpersonal creation of meaning through practical engagement in a social world. Heidegger's phenomenology, therefore, as Bracken goes on to describe in Section II of this book, provides the theoretical framework for an alternative approach to trauma management, one which in being interpersonal rather than intrapsychic, and social rather than individual in orientation, is better suited to the needs of very many victims of trauma, particularly those in the non-Western world.

Others have marked the conflict of paradigms between Western and non-Western models of therapy. Bracken discusses the work of Roland Littlewood and Arthur Kleinman, for example. Littlewood and Kleinman are both psychiatrists and anthropologists rather than philosophers. The distinctive contribution of philosophy, Bracken suggests, is a kind of ground-clearing exercise. And ground-clearing, particularly of the radical conceptual kind offered by philosophy, is important in psychiatry. As Bracken describes, it opens up space for alternative voices; and many of the worst abuses of psychiatry – political, commercial and, indeed, therapeutic – have arisen through one voice coming to shout so loudly as to exclude all others.

But philosophy, as Section III of Bracken's book amply illustrates, also offers a positive agenda for change. Bracken is careful to emphasize that, in contrast to earlier critics of the 'Western' model of psychiatry, it is no part of his brief to invent a new therapy. Yet the model of practice to which his philosophy leads is a new model, nonetheless. Bracken and his colleague Phil Thomas have coined the phrase 'postpsychiatry' for this model. Postpsychiatry incorporates evidence, individual therapy, and impersonal diagnostic categories, the tools of traditional medical psychiatry. But postpsychiatry de-centres these tools of traditional psychiatry and instead foregrounds questions of values, social contexts and, perhaps most important of all, personal meanings.

Postpsychiatry is a timely development in the UK. We are faced, on the one hand, with a new Mental Health Act, Part II of which, if our government has its way, threatens to give 'public safety' a loud if not deafening voice. If the Act becomes law, it is hard to see how psychiatry in the UK as traditionally conceived can avoid becoming increasingly defensive, risk-averse, rule-bound and coercive – little different indeed from the 'political psychiatry' of the former USSR. On the other hand, though, this same government has given us a National Service Framework for Mental Health in which the 'user voice' has been given, perhaps for the first time, a central place. Postpsychiatry supplies the theoretical resources for responding in a balanced way to these conflicting voices; and Bracken, as I noted earlier, has been at the forefront of service developments which seek to turn postpsychiatry theory into effective practice.

Is postpsychiatry a new direction for psychiatry? Well, in focusing psychiatry on social context and personal meanings, it is certainly a new direction for psychiatry at the start of the twenty-first century. For the 1990s – as 'the decade of the brain' – was the fulfilment, the vindication indeed, of a century of scientific effort to understand the causes of mental disorder. Even psychoanalysis, though capable of hermeneutic reconstruction, was conceived originally by Sigmund Freud and has continued to be largely practised within a causal-scientific framework. And the key advances at the end of the twentieth century in understanding the causes of mental disorder have all been in the 'hard' sciences of genetics, brain imaging, and neuropharmacology.

But, historically, postpsychiatry is also a re-newed direction for psychiatry. For at the start of the twentieth century, no less a figure than the founder of modern scientific psychopathology, the German philosopher and psychiatrist, Karl Jaspers, repeatedly emphasized the importance of meanings, as well as causes, in psychiatry. Jaspers' phenomenology, it is true, was a neo-Kantian development of the intrapsychic phenomenology of Husserl. Bracken's work, as noted above, is importantly different from Jaspers' in being based instead on the interpersonal phenomenology of Heidegger. But Bracken and Jaspers are alike in insisting on the importance of meanings as well as causes in understanding mental distress and disorder.

Bracken and Jaspers are also alike in working at a time of flowering of biological methods in psychiatry. This is no coincidence. Just as it was no coincidence that the 1990s, as the decade of the brain, turned out also to be the decade of philosophy in psychiatry. For scientific advances increase rather than decrease the significance of what Peter Campbell, a historian and service-user cited by Bracken, calls the 'new meanings in (our) most vivid personal experiences'. Important as advances in 'biological' psychiatry have been, they will become increasingly abusive in effect if psychiatrists are led by them to deny that, as Campbell says, 'the content of our crises, particularly those they [psychiatrists] define as psychotic, are real, relevant or of anything but negative value'.

In *Trauma: Culture, Meaning and Philosophy*, Bracken, and the postpsychiatry movement he has helped to establish, offer us a vision of a mature psychiatry in which meanings as well as causes, and hence the humanities as well as the sciences, are the basis of good clinical care.

K. W. M. (Bill) Fulford

Acknowledgements

This book began life as a PhD thesis in philosophy, presented at the University of Warwick. I would like to acknowledge the help and support of my supervisors, Professor K.W. M. Fulford and Dr Miguel de Beistegui. My friends and colleagues Dr Derek Summerfield, Dr Pat Coll and Dr Tony O'Connor read the manuscript at various stages of development and gave invaluable advice. I have discussed many of the issues with Dr Phil Thomas here in Bradford. My partner Dr Joan Giller has been part of the project ever since its origins in our work with the Medical Foundation in Uganda in the late 1980s. Special thanks to her for her love and support over the years and for the spelling corrections.

Patrick J. Bracken

Chapter 1
Introduction

The magic circle

Most of us live our lives with a sense that the world we occupy is meaningful. Stars, planets, trees, land, seas, cities, animals and human beings seem to cohere, and together form some sort of totality. Whether or not we believe in a God, we perceive pattern and sometimes harmony all around us. This sense of underlying coherence and order is the basis of our everyday lives. It provides the matrix in which our relationships, our goals and aspirations, our pleasures and our pains all occur. For many people the meaningfulness of the world is simply inherent and they live their lives without ever having cause to question it. It is somewhat like the chequered board upon which a game of chess is played, a taken-for-granted frame in which pieces have roles and relationships and against which different patterns of play can take place. Many people never have cause to look down and examine the 'ground' upon which they move.

However, there are times when the meaningfulness of the world is withdrawn – situations in which all the elements of our lives are still present but the background sense of coherence retreats. At these times it appears that the chequered board has been removed. The pieces remain in place but their connection to one another becomes arbitrary. These are times when we are confronted with the sense that there is no ground at all beneath our feet and our lives come to lack direction and purpose.

These experiences give rise to emotions that range from anxiety to sheer terror. For some, it is an occasional ordeal, associated with lying awake in the early hours of the morning when the darkness and silence of the world can have the effect of emphasizing our solitude and fragility. Most often this anxiety can be put aside as we get ready for the hustle and bustle of our daytime lives. Some people, however, cannot shed this anxiety as the sun comes up and they live out their days with a continuous feeling of dread. Their lives are not shaped by a taken-for-granted order,

1

but are endlessly threatened by the quicksand of meaninglessness. The sickening feelings that go with this dread insinuate themselves into different aspects of life, undermining relationships, work and ambitions. Such people often seek help from healers of one sort or another.

However, these feelings may also serve as a source of creative inspiration. In confronting the contingency of existence the individual is challenged to examine the 'taken-for-granteds' of his or her life. This can lead to the opening up of new imaginative and artistic paths, renewed religious or political engagement or a deepening of personal relationships. Some of the great artistic achievements of the twentieth century such as the works of Kafka and Beckett have emerged directly from a confrontation with the naked contingency of our situation as human beings.

As will become clear in the chapters that follow, I do not believe that there is one particular reason why some people are affected with this sort of anxiety or dread. However, one thing that does seem clear is that of all the creatures we are aware of, it is human beings alone who face the dread brought on by a struggle with meaning. This is probably because it is often related to an intense awareness of our own mortality and that of those we love. As human beings we are both gifted and burdened with the ability to imagine the reality of death. In his book *Post-traumatic Culture*, Kirby Farrell tells us about how, at the age of nine, he first understood that one day he would die. This realization had a profound effect upon him. He describes how his father, who had lost his parents at a young age, broke the news about the death of a 'grandfatherly neighbour'. The father's dread was communicated to the nine-year-old Farrell:

> That night while my mother was out visiting, I lay in my bed in a state of gathering panic. It wasn't dying that terrified me, it was the idea of not being, of being dead forever. In the wisdom of slang, the idea 'got to' me. A storm of adrenaline shook me. One by one I called up a thousand arguments to save my mind, and one by one they fell to shreds. When I tried to think of religion I realized that I couldn't imagine heaven: I couldn't believe in it. Heaven was a word, something people said to calm each other. The feeling of utter helplessness was as much a shock to me as the idea of imminent death. Finally in a spasm of horror I leapt out of bed and ran to my father in the kitchen. I was sweating anguish, leaking tears, and I couldn't talk. And the fear was contagious. In his brusque confusion I felt my father's own invisible, helpless fear.
>
> (Farrell 1998: xi)

Farrell relates how for months after this incident he suffered from anxiety and memories of those first feelings of terror. He connects his reaction to other things happening in his (North American) culture at the time: the end of World War II and the war in Korea, the rising threat of the Soviet Union and the reality of the H-bomb. The anxiety associated with these events served as the backdrop for his own coming to terms with death and nothingness. He recounts this story at the beginning of his book and explains its importance:

> I bring up this story because it illustrates so plainly what can happen when, for whatever reason, we blunder outside the magic circle of everyday life. Natural catastrophe or human violence readily breaks the circle, but under the right conditions any pile up of stresses, any mortal terror, can do it. In trauma, terror overwhelms not just the self, but the ground of the self, which is to say our trust in the world.
>
> (Farrell 1998: xii)

In the course of his book, Farrell traces the way in which trauma became a central motif in various cultural narratives (films, novels and other works) of the 1990s. This echoed a similar process at the end of the nineteenth century when the clinical concept of traumatic neurosis was first developed. Like the Renaissance conception of 'the world as a stage', the notion of trauma has come to serve as a cultural trope that expresses many of the concerns and fears of our time. In this book, I shall be mainly concerned with the question of meaning and how it is sometimes lost from our lives. Most of the text concerns the frameworks and assumptions we use to understand this phenomenon. However, I also focus on the specific issue of trauma, as I believe that, in certain situations, the experience of horror calls into question the basic order of the world. For Farrell, trauma is both a clinical syndrome and a 'strategic fiction that a complex, stressful society is using to account for a world that seems threateningly out of control' (1998: 2). In the following pages, I hope to show the links between these two ways of understanding trauma.

I am struck by Farrell's image of the 'magic circle of everyday life'. By presenting the intelligibility of our world as something like a magic circle he conveys a sense of how wonderful and mysterious the fact of meaningfulness actually is. It may seem unusual to think about the basic order of reality in terms of 'magic'. But it is this sense of order in the world which gives rise to our deepest feelings of awe and wonder. In turn, these feelings inspire religious, scientific and philosophical inquiry. However, the idea of a magic circle also connotes a feeling of fragility and precariousness. It is not to be taken for granted. What happens if we step outside? This work is an attempt to explore the magic circle from a number of directions, it is about some of the different ways we have attempted to understand and respond to the phenomenon of meaning and its withdrawal: philosophical, medical, and sociological.

In my work as a psychiatrist I have come to believe that approaching the problem of meaning and its loss (and mental illness more generally) from a narrow medical perspective is fraught with dangers. Framing problems with our thoughts, emotions, behaviours and relationships in a medical idiom can sometimes be helpful (in the short term at least) but it can also prove limiting and destructive. In recent years, historians, anthropologists, philosophers and service-users themselves have been at pains to point out that psychiatric classification systems do not hold some universal truth about madness or distress. In reality, most psychiatric diagnoses are nothing more than a particular way of formulating and naming a person's problems. On occasions this can be beneficial, as a means whereby a person in chaos is given a framework that can assist in reordering his or her world. It can also allow an individual to shed some responsibility for his/her suffering and behaviour. It gets health professionals and others involved and offers a set of therapeutic options.

However, there is also a downside to diagnosis and the medical framing of distress. It can cover up as well as illuminate the reasons for our pain and suffering. It is often presented to patients as 'the truth' of their condition and serves to silence other possibilities. Psychiatric diagnosis is often little more than a simplification of a complex reality and by formulating an individual's experiences in terms of pathology it can be profoundly disempowering and stigmatizing. Fulford (1994) has used an approach derived from linguistic philosophy to highlight the prevalence of, and significance of, value judgements within psychiatric classifications. He argues that these judgements are not simply a 'nuisance' that can be cleared away through the adoption of ever more empirical scientific classifications. Instead they are at the heart of the psychiatric enterprise:

> Instead of . . . being a mark of deficiency, the evaluative connotations of mental illness are shown to reflect the properties (the logical properties) of its constituent symptoms (such as anxiety) and to reflect these properties as faithfully as the more descriptive connotations of physical illness reflect the corresponding (logical) properties of its constituent symptoms (such as pain).
>
> (Fulford 1994: 219)

Fulford draws a number of conclusions from this. Perhaps most germane to our discussion here is his emphasis on the importance of the patient's experience of illness. This experience is not something secondary to the scientific view of the patient's disorder: rather, it has a validity and an importance of its own. In an approach to mental illness that identifies the centrality of issues of value, the patient's account of his/her own position also becomes central. Like Fulford, I believe that we need a greater sense of humility in the face of our patients' own understanding of their worlds and an increased ability to help people in distress without undermining this understanding by imposing our own. Fulford also argues that in pushing psychiatry towards a confrontation with these issues, philosophy has a vital role to play in the future of the discipline (alongside other discourses such as anthropology, sociology and history). If we do not take these issues seriously we are in danger of ending up like a person walking through the countryside at night with only the beam of a torch to light up the way. While there are trees, fields, mountains and streams all around, we are unable to see these all at once with our single beam of light. We would find it arrogant to assert that the countryside consisted of what showed up through the light of the torch alone. Further sources of illumination are obviously needed if the countryside as a whole is to come into view. In the next section of this introduction I shall outline the background to this book: its genesis in my own clinical work with victims of violence. After that, I shall outline the subjects covered in the three sections.

The philosophy and politics of meaning and memory

This book is, in essence, a discussion of the relationships between meaning, culture and mental illness. I draw on philosophy in an attempt to highlight some of the assumptions we use to understand these relationships. My interest in this area emerged from my work as a psychiatrist in the East African country of Uganda during the years 1987–1991, and my continuing involvement as an occasional consultant for the NGO (non-governmental organization) SCF evaluating projects in West Africa and elsewhere.[1] I worked in Uganda for the Medical Foundation for the Care of Victims of Torture on a project partly funded by the International Secretariat of Amnesty International. The aim of this project was to provide medical and psychotherapeutic help to Ugandans who had suffered torture at the hands of the regimes of Milton Obote and Idi Amin. In Uganda I was challenged by stories of both unimaginable suffering and awe-inspiring resilience. During my time in the country I became increasingly dissatisfied with Western psychiatric models of distress and suffering. They appeared inappropriate in many of the situations in which I found myself. They were too individualistic and 'mentalistic' and seemed to pay little attention to the importance of social context, economics and culture (Bracken et al. 1995). Talking with villagers at medical clinics, traditional healing centres, political meetings and many other places in Uganda convinced me that any understanding of the way in which people experienced and reacted to the suffering of war had to involve a social and cultural perspective as a *central* dimension. I was also horrified by the simplistic models of counselling and therapy which were being imported by Western agencies. My unease led to a search to understand the assumptions underlying concepts such as PTSD in an attempt to delineate both their relevance and their limitations.

In many conflict and post-conflict situations there is currently a great deal of interest on behalf of governments and NGOs in providing help for people with the suffering and memory of violence. On the one hand, many 'psychosocial' projects have been established to help individuals 'process' the various traumas of war and violence. The majority of these work with the assumptions of psychiatry and psychology outlined in Section I of this book and provide therapy, counselling and sometimes medication for those identified as victims. On the other hand, 'truth commissions' of various types have been established in order that the memories of suffering be brought into the open. While these have largely been framed in terms of human rights and questions of justice, they are usually presented as setting out to achieve on the social level what the psychosocial projects do on an individual level: they are also about 'processing' the experiences of war and violence. I believe that both types of endeavour work with certain assumptions (most often unacknowledged) about the nature of memory and truth. These assumptions arise largely from Western discourses such as psychology and human rights. I believe also that serious problems arise when these assumptions are used in non-Western settings. I do not claim to have all the answers to these problems. There is clearly a need for others to bear witness and offer support to individuals and communities who have suffered war and violence. There is a need for help with rebuilding economies and infrastructures. However, decades of experience from development work (with very mixed results) should alert us to the dangers of inserting non-indigenous frameworks and priorities into situations where communities are attempting to rebuild their lives and ways of life.

I discussed above my belief that the way in which we experience our world as meaningful is a source of wonder. Most cultures have grappled with this wonder and mystery through a spiritual idiom. Until the twentieth century most people living in Western cultures believed in religious answers to questions about death and the meaning of life. They understood themselves in terms of souls seeking salvation. In his book *Rewriting the Soul: Multiple Personality and the Sciences of Memory* (1995), the philosopher Ian Hacking argues that scientific understandings of ourselves have come to replace religion in Western thought. In particular, the notion of 'soul' has been replaced by a focus on memory.

We no longer seek the truth about the nature of the soul and debate about the proper path towards salvation. We no longer understand moral behaviour in terms of a relationship with the Divine. Instead, we understand ourselves as creatures whose nature lies in the ways in which our brains are wired and our memories stored. Hacking looks in detail at the concept of multiple personality disorder (like PTSD a recent addition to the nosology of psychiatry) and debates about the reality or otherwise of 'false memory'. He argues that these debates could only occur in a society where there was a shared belief that memory was a 'thing' open to scientific investigation. In relation to the sciences of memory, Hacking advances four theses. These are worth quoting in full:

1. The sciences of memory were new in the latter part of the nineteenth century, and with them came new kinds of truths-or-falsehoods, new kinds of facts, new objects of knowledge.
2. Memory, already regarded as a criterion of personal identity, became a scientific key to the soul, so that by investigating memory (to find out its facts) one would conquer the spiritual domain of the soul and replace it by a surrogate, knowledge about memory.
3. The facts that are discovered in this or that science of memory are a surface knowledge; beneath them is the depth knowledge that there are facts about memory to be found out.
4. Subsequently, what would previously have been debates on the moral and spiritual plane took place at the level of factual knowledge. These political debates all presuppose and are made possible by this depth knowledge.

(Hacking 1995: 198)

Hacking's point is well made. Increasingly, Western societies understand the impact of violence and other types of suffering and formulate questions about responsibility and morality through the sciences of memory and psychology. Most non-Western societies deal with these issues very differently, most often through a mixture of religious, spiritual and political ideas and practices.

Writing about the ways in which Mayan Indians have coped with their terrible experiences of violence during and after Guatemala's long civil war, the anthropologist Patricia Foxen argues that ideas such as 'human rights', 'memory' and 'trauma' are deeply problematic. While Mayan experiences can be (and often are) framed through these concepts, at best these accounts are a distorted version of reality and of questionable validity. She writes:

The politico-legal instrumentality of the human rights concept – based in a broader Western discourse on individualism and rationality – often

veils the untidiness, complexity and cultural agency through which
people experience, interpret and remember the past. The notion of
individual memory as conceptualised by human rights projects often
assumes that individual narratives of the past represent coherent stories
and truths; in documenting abuses, events, places and times, victims
and perpetrators must be neatly categorized in order for stories to make
sense, to have an outcome and a purpose.

(Foxen 2000: 359)

I have already mentioned some of the aims of this book. While my focus is
on meaning, culture and trauma, I am also seeking to question some of
the underlying assumptions of Western psychiatry and psychology. By
taking the reader through some of the current discourse on trauma I hope
to make clear how these assumptions work, both in theory and practice.
My aim is not to disprove any particular theory or deny the efficacy of any
particular form of therapy but to demonstrate that this discourse only
works when we accept a certain set of suppositions about the nature of
human reality and meaning. I identify these suppositions as Cartesianism,
and I hope to encourage greater caution about the relevance of this
discourse to people from cultures that operate with different cosmologies,
ontologies and ways of life.

However, the book is not just about the export of Western psychiatry
to the developing world or its use with non-European communities living
in the West. I am also exploring why Western societies have become so
focused on the issue of trauma in recent years. I look at the phenomenon
of postmodernity to ask if the cultural shift from spiritual ways of understanding ourselves and the decline of other meta-narratives have left us, in
Western societies, with a specific vulnerability with regard to the meaning,
order and purpose of our lives. I also ask whether our current ways of
dealing with the sequelae of trauma and problems with meaning through
psychiatry and other technical forms of psychological intervention are the
most appropriate; whether in fact, this 'technicalization' of the problem of
meaning might actually be making the situation worse.

Three approaches to meaning: psychiatric, phenomenological and postmodern

In the rest of this chapter I shall survey the themes covered in the three
sections of the book. At the heart of this work is an encounter with the
work of the German philosopher Martin Heidegger (1889–1976). I want to
show the relevance of Heidegger's philosophy to contemporary concerns
within psychiatry and psychology. I have found this philosophy helpful in
my endeavours to understand and challenge some of the assumptions

upon which our theories and therapeutic interventions are based. Although undoubtedly abstruse at times, Heidegger's thought is a powerful antidote to the dominance of Cartesianism in the humanities and the human sciences. Hopefully, the relevance of his thought to our concern with meaning and its loss will become clear. However, Heidegger's philosophy is at best a sort of clearing operation. His critique opens up a space in which new ways of understanding ourselves and our difficulties can be developed. I shall argue that while his work generates important questions we need to seek answers elsewhere.

Meaning and psychiatry

Before dealing specifically with Heidegger, I shall look in some detail – in Section I (Chapters 2, 3 and 4) – at the prevailing understanding of meaning and trauma within psychiatry. Trauma has become a cardinal theme in psychiatry and clinical psychology in recent years. Debates about traumatic stress are now centre stage in the world of mental health and therapy:

> . . . the study of trauma has become the soul of psychiatry: The devel-
> opment of posttraumatic stress disorder (PTSD) as a diagnosis has
> created an organized framework for understanding how people's
> biology, conceptions of the world, and personalities are inextricably
> intertwined and shaped by experience. The PTSD diagnosis has reintro-
> duced the notion that many 'neurotic' symptoms are not the result of
> some mysterious, well-nigh inexplicable, genetically based irrationality,
> but of people's inability to come to terms with real experiences that have
> overwhelmed their capacity to cope.
>
> (van der Kolk and McFarlane 1996: 4)

Many practitioners in this area understand post-traumatic problems as arising from a destabilizing effect on the meaningfulness of the victim's world (Meichenbaum 1997; Epstein 1991; Janoff-Bulman 1992; McCann and Pearlman 1990; Lifton 1988; Magomed-Eminov 1997). Therapy is usually directed at restoring a sense of order and purpose in the person's life in the wake of horror. This approach does not start from a philo-sophical sense of wonder but from a need to act, to intervene. It simply takes background intelligibility for granted and directs attention at situa-tions in which there is a problem with meaning.

In this section I shall focus mainly on trauma and its sequelae but, in reality, all of psychiatry is concerned with meaning in one way or another. Many patients with recurrent depression, anxiety or psychotic states grapple with similar questions at some stage. In my opinion, if trauma is the 'soul' of current psychiatry it is because it provides a nexus for larger

contemporary debates about meaning, memory, selfhood and responsibility. I shall discuss the work of the American psychologist Louis Sass. In
later pages in his writing, Sass deals not with trauma, but with various
aspects of psychotic experience (Sass 1990, 1992a). In his beautiful book
*Madness and Modernism: Insanity in the Light of Modern Art, Literature
and Thought* (1992b), Sass presents psychosis both as an encounter with
the intelligibility of reality and as a coming to terms with the contingency
and fragility of the self in the modern world. He points to a resonance
between the struggles of patients diagnosed as schizophrenic and those of
modern artists, writers and philosophers. He notes that many of the most
creative and imaginative minds of the twentieth century had experiences
which could be labelled mental illness.

As a psychologist, Sass is an exception. His approach to psychotic
experience, encountering it as something to be explored and illuminated
by reference to philosophy, art and literature, is very much outside the
dominant paradigm. In the main, psychiatry and psychology encounter a
breakdown in meaning as a scientific problem. As we shall see, cognitive
approaches are currently very popular. These present meaning as
something generated within individual minds through the interaction of
personal 'schemas' with sensory experience. This is understood to be
something amenable to causal explanation and scientific investigation. In
their 1996 book *Mind, Meaning and Mental Disorder: The Nature of
Causal Explanation in Psychology and Psychiatry* Derek Bolton and
Jonathan Hill made a strong case for regarding meaning as something to
be explained causally, albeit with a modified notion of causality. I shall
engage with their ideas later in the book. Their work is essentially an
attempt to provide a philosophical grounding for cognitivism in
psychology and psychiatry. In his foreword to their work, the cognitivist
psychologist Chris Brewin welcomes their attempt to provide philosophical support for the sort of work he is involved with and he
summarizes their arguments:

> The divide between the biological and the psychosocial approach to
> mental illness is shown to be profoundly misleading – instead, Bolton
> and Hill argue, the divide is between intentional explanations and non-
> intentional explanations. According to intentional explanations,
> symptoms arise because normally functioning biological and psycho-
> logical systems are attempting to deal with information that is either
> internally inconsistent or is inconsistent with the person's goals.
> According to non-intentional explanations, the biological or psycho-
> logical systems are themselves malfunctioning, probably as a result of
> some disease process. Both types of explanation may apply at different
> times, and both are equally 'scientific'.
>
> (Brewin 1996: vi)

In other words, Bolton and Hill argue that because biological and psychological 'systems' deal with information and 'intentionality' they can be analysed in similar ways. From this perspective, the meaningfulness of our lives shows up as 'information' and is open to scientific analysis in the same way that biological systems can be analysed. Bolton and Hill assert that because in their framework the psychological and the biological have similar properties they have effectively taken us beyond dualism and Cartesianism. I shall argue against this and attempt to show that in spite of their assertion to the contrary, cognitivism continues to work with an essentially Cartesian understanding of human reality. As such, it is a limited attempt to grasp the way in which we experience our worlds as meaningful. However, I want to be clear: in this book my aim is not to argue that cognitivism and its assumptions are wrong. I simply want to demonstrate, through an analysis of one area of concern (trauma and its sequelae) that there are other (equally valid) ways of understanding ourselves and our problems. My task in the first section of the book is to show that there *are* assumptions at work and to attempt to sketch their nature.

Meaning and phenomenology

In Section II (Chapters 5, 6, 7 and 8), I turn to the world of continental philosophy and the work of Heidegger and his psychiatric colleague Medard Boss (1903–1990). While Heidegger did not write about trauma as such, I believe that his philosophical approach to the question of meaning and its withdrawal offers an important alternative to cognitive approaches. Readers without any prior knowledge of continental philosophy might find parts of this section somewhat difficult. In many ways, Cartesianism has become the 'common sense' of Western culture. The words and phrases we commonly use to describe ourselves and our thinking incorporate its assumptions and, in a world dominated by computers and information systems of different kinds, attempting to think about 'mind' without using a cognitivist idiom is always going to be an uphill struggle. Heidegger's use of words seems strange at times and off-putting. In his introduction to Heidegger, George Steiner writes:

> Much of what Heidegger says is simultaneously obvious and arcane. In order to clarify and, at the same time, to make problematic – and therefore salient – the existential fabric of everyday experience, the seamless texture of being which metaphysics has idealized or scorned, Heidegger welds language into a kind of violent ordinariness. He twists and compacts the sinews of vocabulary and grammar into resistant, palpable nodes. The resultant 'anti-rhetoric' is both highly technical and crassly innocent. As are Expressionist canvases or action paintings, with

their thick swirls and stabs of pigment. [sic] The analogy here is a genuine one. Heidegger is striving to get language and his reader inside the actual world, he is trying to make luminous and self-revealing the obstinate opaqueness of matter.

(Steiner 1978: 84–85)

Heidegger's work was very much an attempt to get beyond the thinking of Descartes and other philosophers of the Enlightenment, and he stands as one of the most important inspirations for European philosophy in the second half of the twentieth century. His work is the central reference point for existentialism, hermeneutics and postmodern approaches. His work was on a vast scale, and some of his papers are still appearing in the *Gesamtausgabe*, the collected edition of his writings. He remains a controversial figure in European philosophy. The fact that he became a member of the Nazi party in the 1930s, and his continued silence on the Holocaust after the war, point to a need for caution with regard to some of the answers he gave to the questions raised by his philosophy.[2] I do not wish to enter the many disputes about the proper interpretation of Heidegger's work. I am particularly sympathetic to the approach of Hubert Dreyfus, widely acknowledged as being largely responsible for introducing Heidegger's thought to this current generation of philosophers, particularly those in North America (Wrathall and Malpas 2000). My reading of *Being and Time* is guided by his well-known commentary (Dreyfus 1991).

Heidegger's aim in *Being and Time* is to examine the question of being, the central preoccupation of traditional Western metaphysics, in a completely new light. While the notion of 'being' might sound vague, Dreyfus maintains that 'what Heidegger has in mind when he talks about being is the intelligibility correlative with our everyday background practices'. In other words: 'to raise the question of being (is) to make sense of our ability to make sense of things' (Dreyfus 1991: 10).

The question of being is not about the nature of things in the world such as objects and thoughts; it is the question of how the world makes sense for us, of how it is meaningful. According to Heidegger, the meaningfulness of the world is primary. In other words, we experience the world first and foremost as a whole and only then do we encounter particular things within that world. Entities show up as meaningful for us only against a background context. But this background cannot be generated by a simple listing of things. The point is that we experience the things of our world as related or as contrasted, but always as 'holding together' in some way. Unlike the analytic approach of psychiatry and psychology, whose priority is explanation, Heidegger wants to provoke a sense of wonder in regard to this issue. He distinguishes two areas of inquiry, which he labels 'ontological' and 'ontic'. Ontological inquiry refers to the question of being (the background 'holding together') while ontic enquiry refers to a concern with entities and facts about them (Heidegger 1962: 31). Ontological inquiry has to be undertaken in a way different from any type of ontic enquiry. Being has to be 'exhibited in a way of its own'. Thus, for Heidegger, the question of meaning cannot, and should not, be framed as a scientific issue.[3] The meaning of being is simply not 'something' that can be grasped through a causal framework. In fact, it is not a 'thing' at all and it requires a very different type of understanding to that provided by science. For Heidegger, in *Being and Time*, the path to understanding the meaning of being was through an analysis of the only entity for which this question arose: human being.

Heidegger was a student of the founder of phenomenology[4], Edmund Husserl, and his philosophical enterprise was essentially an attempt to reorient phenomenology away from what Heidegger saw as Husserl's misguided focus on 'pure' internal consciousness towards understanding human 'being' as 'being-in-the-world', grounded always in a life-world shaped by culture and history. Heidegger put hermeneutics[5] at the centre of his approach to phenomenology. Through his influence on Hans-Georg Gadamer, Paul Ricoeur and others, Heidegger has inspired a whole series of interpretive positions in the social sciences (Geertz 1973). These emphasize the importance of life-world and the primacy of interpretation. However, the phenomenological approach has been virtually absent from recent discussions of trauma and in other areas of psychiatry (apart from psychotherapy, discussed in Chapter 6) only a very 'Husserlian' form of phenomenology has had a presence (Bracken 1999). In this book, I wish to highlight the importance of Heidegger's insights in the world of mental health. However, following Dreyfus, I shall also point to what I consider to be major contradictions and limitations of Heidegger's position as spelt out in *Being and Time*.

Meaning and postmodernity

In Section III (Chapters 10 and 11), I shall look at some of the implications of postmodernity for the issue of meaning and mental illness. The term 'postmodernity' is often used to refer to a contemporary social, cultural and political *condition*, something we simply find ourselves in the midst of. I wish to separate this from a different and more positive use of the term as a particular *way of reflecting* upon the world and our place within it. This is a concept of postmodernity as:

> . . . a form of reflection upon and a response to the accumulating signs of the limits and limitations of modernity. Postmodernity as a way of

living with the doubts, uncertainties and anxieties which seem increasingly to be a corollary of modernity, the inescapable price to be paid for
the gains, the benefits and the pleasures, associated with modernity.

(Smart 1993: 12)

I shall suggest that recent cultural developments in the Western world
have created a situation where the meaningfulness of our lives is systematically called into question. We live in the midst of a very creative and
dynamic, but also very fragile, culture. From an economic point of view,
postmodern societies are dependent for their vitality on ever-increasing
patterns of consumption. This requires a continuing incitement to identify
new desires and needs. Products are increasingly sold, not for their use-
value but for what they symbolize about a way of life. We are tutored by
marketing and the media to define ourselves in terms of the food we eat,
the clothes we wear, the holidays we buy and the style of our homes and
gardens. There is an economic drive to continually rewrite the narratives
and meta-narratives of our lives. Even religion has become 'commodified'
in a sort of new age spiritual consumerism.

On one level, we experience this as a liberation – a shedding of
oppressive stereotypes and a casting off of stifling identities. But, on
another level, there is clearly a loss, because it is these strong religious,
cultural and political narratives that have – until now at least – provided
the ground upon which we achieve a sense of meaning and purpose. In
this book, I shall link the economic and cultural shift to an intense form of
consumer capitalism and postmodernity with our contemporary
experience of trauma, distress and alienation. On a more optimistic note, I
shall argue that insights from postmodern thought have important
positive implications for how we *respond* to trauma, both in the context of
postmodern cultures and with victims of violence from other cultures
where a strong communal cosmology remains in place.

However, I'm afraid that if the reader is looking for a new theory of
trauma or a new therapeutic technique in this work then he/she will be
disappointed. The reader will find few certainties in this book. What I
hope they will find is an invitation to questioning, a solicitation to wonder.
Philosophy cannot tell us what to do clinically, but by challenging assumptions and accepted ways of thinking about ourselves and our distress it can
encourage a deepened sensibility with regard to suffering and with this an
opening up of new therapeutic possibilities.[6]

SECTION I
Trauma, meaning and psychiatry

Chapter 2
Enlightenment, psychiatry and the nature of mind

In this section (Chapters 2, 3 and 4) I will be discussing the concept of PTSD and how the prevailing discourse on trauma has turned to cognitive psychology to frame its understanding of how meaning is undermined in post-traumatic reactions. My primary aim in this section is not to give the reader a detailed overview of contemporary work on trauma but to emphasize the underlying philosophical assumptions at work. I will begin, in Part I of this chapter, by discussing the emergence of psychiatry from the culture and thought of the European Enlightenment and I will attempt to show how a particular set of philosophical principles came to guide its development in the twentieth century. In Part II, I will go on to argue that recent developments in cognitive psychology have incorporated these principles. In the next chapter, I turn to the discourse on trauma itself and show how it has worked to deal with the question of meaning within the parameters set by modern psychiatry and psychology. In Chapter 4, I will discuss the successes and limitations of this approach.

I The European Enlightenment

A central concern of the European Enlightenment was the importance of reason and its place in human affairs. Finding a path to true knowledge and certainty became the major issue for thinkers during the Enlightenment and epistemology (theories of knowledge, truth and certainty) became the central concern of philosophy. A guiding theme was the quest to replace religious revelation, and systems of knowledge from the past, with reason and science as the path to truth. As Norman Hampson argues:

> The cultural horizon of most educated men in western Europe in the early seventeenth century was dominated by two almost unchallenged sources of authority: scripture and the classics. Each in its own way perpetuated the idea that civilization had degenerated from a former

17

> Golden Age. The most rational preoccupation for contemporary man
> was, therefore, by the study of the more fortunate ancients to move back
> towards the kind of society, which the latter had known. Recent
> European movements, the Renaissance and the Reformation, had
> reinforced this attitude and enhanced the authority of the sacred texts.
>
> (Hampson 1968: 16)

Enlightenment[1] meant a move from 'darkness' to 'light'. To achieve this,
reason would have boldly to give up its preoccupation with those things
handed down in tradition. The German philosopher Immanuel Kant
(1724–1804) was one of the pre-eminent voices of the Enlightenment. He
declared that:

> Enlightenment is man's emergence from his self-incurred immaturity.
> Immaturity is the inability to use one's understanding without the
> guidance of another. This immaturity is called 'self-incurred' if its cause
> is not lack of understanding but lack of resolution and courage to use it
> without the guidance of another. The motto of Enlightenment is
> therefore: *Sapere aude!* Have courage to use your own understanding!
>
> (Kant 1992: 305)

The other preoccupation of European thought emerging from the
Enlightenment, particularly on the continent, was with the human self and
its depths. European thinkers became concerned with the 'inner voice'
and the structures of subjectivity. Robert Solomon points out that in the
work of Kant in particular, this preoccupation attained its full force. Kant's
philosophy was an attempt to vindicate the power of reason. He did this,
not through an analysis of religious texts or through a look back to the
ancient Greeks, but via a detailed critical examination of reason itself. His
focus was inwards, on the nature of human experience. On what basis do
we make judgements about space and time? What principles are 'built
into' our understanding? In many ways, in Kant's philosophy the structures of subjectivity become the entire subject matter of philosophy. For
him:

> The self is not just another entity in the world, but in an important sense
> it creates the world, and the reflecting self does not just know itself, but
> in knowing itself knows all selves, and the structures of any and every
> possible self.
>
> (Solomon 1988: 6)

My thesis is that the disciplines of psychology and psychiatry only became
possible in a cultural framework substantially influenced by these
Enlightenment and post-Enlightenment preoccupations. These disciplines

represented a search for scientific accounts of the mind and its disorders. They depended on theories of the self and behaviour, which would *explain* human actions and so allow for technical interventions to be made on a rational basis. The structures of the self were to be revealed and defined. As Jerome Levin writes:

> In premodern conceptualisations, the self had been seen as safely coherent and enduring, deriving its stability from its relationship with God, but now something else was required as a cement. The old verities were no longer certain, and the unity of the self, itself, was now problematical.
>
> (Levin 1992: 16)

The Enlightenment gave rise to new questions and new ways of answering. In the modern world the question of meaning would no longer be left to God and his prophets and priests. Science and rationality were to take hold of this question and psychiatry was to have a central role; likewise with madness. On a more practical level, with its focus on reason and order, the Enlightenment spawned an era in which society sought to rid itself of all 'unreasonable' elements. As the historian Roy Porter writes:

> The Enlightenment endorsed the Greek faith in reason ('I *think*, therefore I am,' Descartes had claimed). And the enterprise of the age of reason, gaining authority from the mid-seventeenth century onwards, was to criticize, condemn and crush whatever its protagonists considered to be foolish or unreasonable. All beliefs and practices which appeared ignorant, primitive, childish or useless came to be readily dismissed as idiotic or insane, evidently the products of stupid thought-processes, or delusion and daydream. And all that was so labelled could be deemed inimical to society or the state – indeed could be regarded as a menace to the proper workings of an orderly, efficient, progressive, rational society.
>
> (Porter 1987: 14–15)

In Michel Foucault's account, the emergence of the institutions in which 'unreasonable' people were to be housed was not in itself a 'progressive', or medical, venture. It was simply, and crudely, an act of social exclusion. He coined the term 'The Great Confinement' (Foucault 1971). Furthermore, he argued that it was only when such people had been both excluded and brought together that they became subject to the 'gaze' of medicine. According to Foucault, doctors were originally involved in these institutions in order to treat physical illness and to offer moral guidance. They were not there as experts in disorders of the mind. As time went on, the medical profession came to dominate in these institutions and doctors began to order and classify the inmates in more systematic ways. Roy Porter writes:

> Indeed, the rise of psychological medicine was more the consequence than the cause of the rise of the insane asylum. Psychiatry could flourish once, but not before, large numbers of inmates were crowded into asylums.
>
> (Porter 1987: 17)

Medical superintendents of asylums gradually became psychiatrists, but they did not start out as such. Alongside the increasing hegemony of psychiatrists, the concept of mental illness became accepted. In other words, in this account, the profession of psychiatry and its associated technologies of diagnosis and treatment only became possible in the institutional arena opened up by an original act of social rejection. Perhaps this explains some of the stigma which has been attached to psychiatry and its patients in spite of the former's protestations of its scientific credentials. Historically, psychiatry emerged to label those who had *already* been rejected and thus its diagnoses quickly became symbols of rejection in themselves. While a number of psychiatrists and historians have questioned various aspects of Foucault's account and it has become increasingly clear that the story of psychiatry has varied greatly from country to country (Foucault's focus was upon developments in France), nevertheless there is a general acceptance that his rejection of a simple 'progressivist' version of psychiatry's development is justified (Gordon, 1990).

    Thus, according to Porter, Foucault and others, on the practical level of how society responded to 'unreasonable' people, the Enlightenment marked a major turning point. With reason replacing religion as the guide to social progress, such people (including those regarded as insane) came to be seen as an obstacle to progress and were to be systematically excluded. However, the Enlightenment also engendered new ways of thinking about the mind and about meaning and madness. These took origin from the work of the French philosopher René Descartes (1596–1650). In the next section, I explore some of Descartes' ideas about the mind and the nature of thought. In many ways these ideas are now part of our 'common-sense' understanding of ourselves but we shall see that they have also influenced the sort of phenomenology developed by Edmund Husserl (1859–1938), which, through its influence on the philosopher and psychiatrist Karl Jaspers (1883–1969), has had a major impact on twentieth century psychiatry.

The Cartesian understanding of human reality

I will refer to the 'Cartesian tradition' at a number of points in the book. My use of this term is indebted to Hubert Dreyfus's discussion of 'Cartesianism' in his *Being-in-the-World: A Commentary on Heidegger's Being and Time* (Dreyfus 1991). I am aware that there are different interpretations of Descartes and my references to his work will not be extensive. However, many of the philosophers quoted in this book, including Heidegger, have seen their work as being in direct opposition to a Cartesian account of human reality. It is important therefore to say something about what this account entails. A central theme of the book involves an attempt to think about mind, meaning and distress from outside the current frameworks of psychology and psychiatry. Before we can get outside we need to understand the assumptions upon which these frameworks are built.

Reason and certainty

The central philosophical problem for Descartes was the question of certainty: how can we be certain that our internal mental representations give us an accurate account of the external world? His answer was to propose a method of systematic reflection upon the contents of the mind and through this to separate what was clear and obviously accurate from what was uncertain and vague. Descartes was impressed by the certainty and clarity of mathematics and saw mathematics as the key to progress in the rest of science and philosophy. In his *Meditations on First Philosophy* (published in Latin in 1641) he argued that by way of systematically doubting everything that was unclear we could eventually reach a situation of certainty with regard to our own existence, the existence of God and the existence and nature of the external world. Even though I can doubt many things there is one idea, reasoned Descartes, which I know always to be true: the fact that I am thinking. I simply cannot be mistaken when I think that I am thinking. In fact, I know that I exist because I know that I am thinking. This has become known as the Cartesian cogito.[2]

With this as his starting point, he went on to argue that by examining our beliefs very carefully we could also be certain that other thoughts were true. While we can be deceived at times by our senses, if we accept that God is good, and 'on our side', there is, according to Descartes, no reason to postulate that he would have set the world up so that we would be *systematically* deceived by our senses. Thus, if we confine ourselves to thoughts and beliefs that are 'clear and distinct' (such as the concepts of mathematics) we can work to avoid error. Our reason or intellect is a gift from God and as long as we use it properly we can use it to avoid mistakes.

For Descartes, certainty is reached by turning away from the world and examining one's own thoughts in isolation. While a 'non-deceiving' God was the ultimate guarantor of truth and certainty, his presence was not essential to his confidence in our ability to clarify our thinking and to separate the clear and distinct thoughts from others. Even in the absence of a guarantor of truth, systematic reflexivity is able to render us better able to account for our thoughts. A central tenet of Cartesianism is therefore a belief in the importance of, and the possibility of, reflexive clarity and in the importance of defining and mapping the ways in which internal representations are ordered and related.

Cartesian dualism: ontological and epistemological

In addition, Cartesianism operates on a fundamental distinction between the 'inner' world of the mind and the 'outer' world with which it is in contact. This separation of the inner and the outer is predicated upon Descartes' ontological separation of the world into two kinds of substance, so-called Cartesian dualism. The term substance is the philo-sophical equivalent of the ordinary word 'thing' (*res*). Descartes separated out the soul from the material body in which it resided. The latter he characterized as follows:

> . . . by body, I understand all that can be terminated by some figure; that can be contained in some place and fill a space in such a way that any other body is excluded from it.
>
> (Descartes 1968:104)

In other words, the body is characterized by the fact that it possesses 'extension'; it is thus *res extensa*. In contrast to this the soul is charac-terized by thought:

> . . . I am therefore, precisely speaking, only a thing which thinks, that is to say, a mind, understanding, or reason, terms whose significance was hitherto unknown to me. I am, however, a real thing, and really existing; but what thing? I have already said it: a thing which thinks.
>
> (Descartes 1968: 105)

The soul, or the self, is thus 'a thing which thinks', a *res cogitans*. While it does not occupy space, Descartes still maintained that it was a substance, a *res*, a thing. This application of the concept of thing or substance, to the self has had major implications. The term substance is usually applied to familiar objects such as trees or chairs. In pre-Enlightenment scholastic philosophy a distinction was made between the attributes of a thing and that within which such attributes resided. The latter was called the *substantia*, that which 'stands beneath' the attributes. The substance, as that in which the attributes or properties of a thing inhere, cannot be readily perceived or described. Nevertheless it is what gives the thing its existence as a singular entity. In the concept of substance used by Descartes, this contrast between the plurality of the attributes and the singleness of that in which they reside is fundamental. When moved to the self, the *res cogitans,* this contrast is maintained, but operates in a somewhat different way. Frederick Olafson formulates this as follows:

> To the attributes of the standard substance or thing, there now correspond the representations or ideas of the things that the self perceives or otherwise thinks about; and to the mysterious nucleus in which those properties were supposed to inhere, there corresponds that in which these representations are contained. It is as though substance in the picture we ordinarily form of it had been turned inside out or, better still, outside in. Indeed, this is not a bad way of understanding the change that has taken place, since to the attribute that a thing like an apple displays to general view, there now corresponds a representation *within* the new kind of substance, but with this difference, that the representation is accessible only to the view from within and cannot be perceived from without at all.
>
> (Olafson 1987: 7)

Thus thoughts, perceptions, beliefs, desires and other mental phenomena are the attributes, or properties, which inhere within the mind. Thought becomes the inner functioning of a substance, which we call a subject (*subjectum*). This subject is in contact with an outside world and has knowledge of it through sensation and through the representations it has of it. The point is that in this Cartesian view the mind becomes something 'self-contained'. It stands outside the world and has a relationship to it. Mind becomes something conceivable apart from and separate from this relation. It knows the world from the outside. Thus, there is an epistemological separation of mind from world.

It is this epistemological separation, based ultimately, as we have seen, on Descartes' ontological dualism, which provides the basis for what is known as the representational theory of mind and thought, concerned as it with the relationship between inner states of mind and outer states of the world. As Dreyfus points out, modern information-processing models of mind and the functionalist philosophies of mind (see below) that go with them are, in essence, updated versions of this approach (Dreyfus 1991: 115). Descartes' epistemological separation also provides the source for the sort of phenomenology developed by Husserl and his followers.

The Cartesian orientation of Husserl's phenomenology and modern psychiatry

Husserl's orientation towards the Cartesian project is overtly positive (the title of one of his major works is *Cartesian Meditations*). His fundamental method of enquiry, which he called 'phenomenological reduction', involved setting aside, or 'bracketing', the existence of an outside world in order to focus in a clear and unbiased way upon the phenomena of consciousness and experience. His aim was to reach what he called the 'transcendental standpoint'.[3] This was to be achieved by a series of 'reductions' which, in turn, were operations performed upon everyday experience with the purpose of isolating the 'pure' consciousness which is obscured as long as it is not separated from the natural world. Like Descartes, Husserl was attempting to elaborate a method of investigation into the experiential world, which was solid and foundational. Louis Sass says:

> Like Descartes' method of doubt, Husserl's approach can be called a
> kind of 'foundationalism': an attempt to discover a realm of indubitable
> and transparent meanings or experiential entities that can provide a firm
> basis on which to build valid knowledge about human existence.
>
> (Sass 1989: 443)

Following Descartes, Husserl's transcendental phenomenology starts with a radical separation between the world of consciousness and the world 'outside' it. However, in some ways Husserl goes a step further than Descartes. His 'bracketing' of the natural world extends to the lived life of the person doing the bracketing. His/her body, history and personality are bracketed along with everything else and become the 'empirical ego'. This is in contrast to the 'transcendental ego' of pure consciousness. In this strategy the empirical ego becomes ranked alongside the objects of the natural world and thus an appropriate domain of scientific enquiry. In this way the end result of Husserl's phenomenology is an endorsement of the project of scientific psychology.[4]

One of the most influential twentieth-century psychiatric texts is Karl Jaspers' *General Psychopathology* (1963). Jaspers worked within the framework of phenomenological psychology developed by Husserl and acknowledges this overtly in the text (1963: 55). As we have seen above, in this theoretical tradition the mind is understood as internal and separate from the world around it. Jaspers also distinguished the form of a mental symptom from its content:

> It is true in describing concrete psychic events we take into account the
> particular contents of the individual psyche, but from the phenomeno-
> logical point of view it is only the form that interests us.
>
> (Jaspers 1963: 59)

This view had an extraordinary influence on European psychiatry. Aubrey Lewis described *General Psychopathology* as 'one of the most important and influential books there are in psychiatry' (quoted by Beaumont 1992). Following Jaspers, twentieth-century psychiatry has continually sought to separate mental phenomena from background contexts. Psychosis and emotional distress are defined in terms of disordered individual experience. Social and cultural factors are, at best, secondary, and may or may not be taken into account (Samson 1995). They are usually understood to influence the content and not the form of psychiatry phenomena. To some extent this orientation results from the fact that most psychiatric encounters occur in hospitals and clinics, with a therapeutic focus on the individual, with drugs or psychotherapy. But it is also because biological, behavioural, cognitive and psychodynamic approaches share a conceptual and therapeutic focus on the individual self.

Cognitivism and Cartesianism

Thus Cartesianism provides an account of the self and thought which has been articulated in different ways through different philosophies. It has, in many ways, come to be taken as 'common sense' within Western cultures. In their book *Mind, Meaning and Mental Disorder: The Nature of Causal Explanation in Psychology and Psychiatry* Derek Bolton and Jonathan Hill argue that Cartesian dualism provided the 'thought space' in which behaviourist psychology emerged. However, they, like most other philosophers, wish to move us beyond both Descartes and behaviourism, and they suggest that cognitive psychology has effectively allowed us to do so. For them, the problem with Cartesian philosophy is its presentation of mental states as 'epistemically private, inaccessible to public observation and verification' (Bolton and Hill 1996: 4). Cognitivism, by making mental states the object of scientific enquiry, is thus seen as being opposed to the Cartesian framework. However, Bolton and Hill appear mainly concerned to surpass *ontological* dualism. They argue that we simply need to 'merge' Cartesian thought and matter and they suggest that cognitivism does this:

> . . . a (or the) defining attribute of Cartesian mind was *thinking*, which is closely linked to representation, meaning, and intentionality, and these are none other than the characteristics of mental states which are essential for the purposes of cognitive explanations of behaviour . . . what was essential to the Cartesian mind is essential also to mind as posited by cognitive-behavioural explanations. This means that the latter will not be satisfied with any definition of mental states that makes them 'material' *as opposed to* 'thoughtful' . . . if mind is going to be identified with the material brain, then the material brain will have to be – like Cartesian mind – a 'thinking substance'.
>
> (Bolton and Hill 1996: 74–75)

Bolton and Hill argue for an approach in which the brain is understood to 'encode' meaning. Because of this the activity of the brain cannot be grasped in terms of traditional notions of causality alone. They propose the existence of 'intentional causality' that comes into play when material systems are involved in 'meaningful' activity, involving the passage and storage of information. Biological and psychological systems are said to exhibit 'intentional causality'. Because of this such systems lend themselves to scientific investigation with the generation of predictive theories. I shall return to the work of Bolton and Hill later in this book, when I present a Heideggerian critique of scientific reductionism. Suffice it to say here that I am not convinced that they genuinely move us away from the Cartesian account of human reality presented above. I tend to agree with Dreyfus that information-processing accounts of mind are still firmly within a Cartesianism framework. While cognitivism does move us away from an *ontological* dualism, it continues to operate with a strong epistemological separation between the mind and the world outside. McCulloch makes this point in his book *The Mind and its World* (1995), in which he argues the case for an *externalist* account of mind. He argues that even if we move beyond the 'immaterialism' involved in Cartesian ontology we are still left with Descartes' separation of the mind from 'its' body and from the world around it. He says that 'vanishingly *little* is settled when immaterialism is rejected' (1995: xii). A similar argument is made by Button et al. in their book *Computers, Minds and Conduct* (1995).

So far in this chapter I have identified Cartesianism with two funda-mental assumptions, which continue to dominate thinking within psychology and psychiatry. These are:

1. an endorsement of methodological individualism and a belief in the possibility of, and the importance of, detached reflection upon the contents of mind;
2. the epistemological acceptance of an a priori separation of mind from world, in which an interior mind relates through representations to an exterior world.

In the next part of the chapter I want to show how a further assumption emerging from the Enlightenment has also come to orient psychiatric thought and practice. This is:

3. a belief in the causal nature of psychological events and a reliance on positivism to guide research and theory formation.

For convenience I will include positivism within the concept of Cartesianism even though, as we shall see in the next section, it is more directly a product of the empirical tradition in scientific and philosophical thought. Mary Hesse's definition of Cartesianism as something based on both rationalist[5] and empiricist principles is close to what I am trying to describe. She says that the assumptions of Cartesianism:

> . . . constitute a picture of science and the world somewhat as follows: there is an external world which can in principle be exhaustively described in scientific language. The scientist, as both observer and language-user, can capture the external facts of the world in propositions that are true if they correspond to the facts and false if they do not.
>
> (Hesse 1980: vii)

In the next section we shall look at the third assumption and the way in which this reliance on positivism has developed in medicine and psychiatry.

Science, positivism and psychiatry

The Enlightenment gave rise to a new orientation within science: a rejection of the 'traditional' Aristotelian[6] ordering of the world and its replacement by a method focused on observation. While both rationalism and empiricism were products of the Enlightenment, empiricism was more dominant in the natural sciences. John Stuart Mill's *System of Logic* (published in 1843) provided the philosophical foundation for empiricism as the ground of all knowledge. Mill advocated the use of natural science methods in the study of human phenomena and said that the 'backward state of the moral sciences' would only be remedied if the 'methods of the physical sciences duly extended and generalized' were applied in them (Mill 1953).

The word 'positivism' comes originally from Auguste Comte's *Cours de Philosophie Positive*.[7] Comte attempted to explore reality through the assessment of facts available to experience. He sought to establish the authority of observation and, like Mill, argued that the methods of the natural sciences were the only properly scientific methods available to researchers in the human or social sciences. Furthermore, science should be seen as a value-free enterprise dealing in objective facts generated by disinterested observation. Since the time of Comte the term 'positivism' has been used to cover a range of philosophical positions. However, Polkinghorne identifies three central themes:

> (1) Metaphysics should be rejected and knowledge confined to what has been experienced or can be experienced.

(2) The adequacy of knowledge increases as it approximates the forms
of explanation that have been achieved by the most advanced sciences.
(3) Scientific explanation is limited to only functional and directional
laws
                                                        (Polkinghorne 1984: 18)

Alongside empiricism and positivism, the nineteenth century also saw the
emergence of naturalism[8]: the belief that all phenomena could be
adequately explained in terms of natural causes and laws without
attributing supernatural, spiritual or moral significance to them. The
anthropologist Deborah Gordon argues this assumption is incorporated
into the way in which Western medicine (what is usually referred to as
'biomedicine') understands itself:

> Biomedical practitioners approach sickness as a natural phenomenon,
> legitimise and develop their knowledge using a naturalist method
> (scientific rationality) and see themselves as practising on nature's
> human representative – the human body.
>
>   (Gordon 1988: 24)

Biomedicine assumes a naturalist epistemology:

> Naturalist truth is not supernatural or spiritual knowledge but the truth
> of matter, of mechanism. 'Truth' is in the accurate explanation of
> material reality, not in the good, or the beautiful, or the spiritual.
> Naturalist knowledge should maintain the separation between culture
> and reality. Culture – symbols and language – are vehicles for knowing;
> they connect the outside reality with the internal knower.
>
> They should leave no trace on the knowledge, that is, they should
> depict rather than constitute . . . Rationality is also separate from
> morality. In fact it is supposed to be stripped of value and to present
> only 'facts'. Truth tells us about how things work 'naturally' not ideolog-
> ically. Finally, ideally truth is beyond time and space – singular,
> universal, eternal, and neutral.
>
>   (Gordon 1988: 30)

Biomedicine incorporates this naturalist epistemology as its 'official'
theory of knowledge, and uses science to provide its criteria of truth. A
combination of naturalism, empiricism and positivism came to dominate
the methodological framework for medicine and the behavioural sciences
such as psychology, and has continued to do so up to the present time.
Hilary Putnam termed it the 'received view' (Putnam 1962). This dominant
system provides epistemological support for experimental designs based
upon empirical data. It constitutes the approved approach to science, and
it is communicated within the social and behavioural sciences through the
primary agencies of disciplinary orthodoxy such as: the standard

textbooks on research, the editorial policies of disciplinary journals and the guidelines for acceptable doctoral dissertations. In the main these call for the use of a methodology based on this approach (Polkinghorne 1984: 60). I shall use the term 'positivism' to broadly denote this 'received view', incorporating empiricism and naturalism.

During the last hundred years much Anglo-American philosophy of science has been devoted to detailed development of the internal logic of natural science. It attained its clearest explanation in the work of the group of philosophers known as the 'Vienna Circle'. Science, they argued, explains events by way of a 'deductive-nomological' method through which theories are accurately deduced from observational data. Theory is stated in the form of universal causal laws, which can be used to predict, as well as explain, events. Through this prediction theories can, in turn, be tested.

Empirical science sought to replace any assumptions or inexplicit links in the process of knowing, with fully explicit observations and fully explicit deductions from these observations. However, as Hume argued in 1739, if all but sense impressions were excluded as sources of knowledge then 'causation' as such does not show up. According to Hume, 'cause' is simply a habit of thought, which people add to the sense data (Hume 1962). Thus the most that we can truly know is that two events have been constantly conjoined in our sense experience. On the basis of our observations alone we cannot know that they will always be so conjoined and that one event causes the other. Philosophers of science committed to the deductive-nomological system had to approach this matter of causation in such a way that it could fit in with their system. To this end they replaced the notion of one event 'resulting' from another with the notion that a certain kind of relationship held between these events. They characterized the kinds of relationship as 'necessary' or 'sufficient'. If a necessary relationship exists between events then the presence of one event is a necessary condition for the presence of a second event. A sufficient relationship can be characterized as follows: 'if A, then B'. B will always occur if A is present. B 'might' occur if A is absent, but it 'must' occur if A is present. In the deductive-nomological system, when a relationship exists between events of a sufficient condition, it is spoken of as a causal relationship or as a causal law, examples of which are abundant in medicine. For instance, if an insulin-dependent diabetic does not receive exogenous doses of insulin regularly then he or she will become comatose.

For positivism, the ability of science to identify such causal relationships through the deductive-nomological type of methodology underlies its predictive force and its explanatory power.[9] These factors in turn explain the success of the natural sciences. If the human sciences were to aspire to such success they too would have to produce deductive-nomological explanations. Within the 'received view' of science, two assumptions are made about the human sciences: first, that observations can be made objectively and that measures can be defined objectively and applied in a precise, replicable fashion; second, that theories can be constructed on the same causal and deterministic basis as in the natural sciences. The ultimate goal of positivism is to provide an objective, empirical and systematic foundation for all knowledge. It is an inherent assumption of positivist philosophy that this is possible. Stemming from this is another basic assumption: that science is progressive. The accumulation of facts about the world leads to an increasingly detailed and informative picture of reality, both natural and human.

This concept of science and knowledge lies at the heart of Western medicine's understanding of itself. In particular, medical research sees itself as attempting to provide a set of value-free techniques that will alleviate pain and suffering by successfully combating disease. It presents itself as disinterested and empirical in its description of the human organism and its diseases, and as steadily progressive in its understanding of the same. Psychiatry, which conceives of itself as a branch of biomedicine, generally follows suit.

Positivism and psychiatry

Since its beginnings in the nineteenth century, psychiatry has been at pains to demonstrate its medical and scientific credentials. In general psychiatric textbooks, an introductory chapter usually contains a brief statement of the positivist nature of psychiatric research and theory. For example, according to Mayer-Gross, Slater and Roth (1960: 24): 'The foundations of psychiatry have to be laid on the ground of the natural sciences.'

Most psychiatrists see themselves as working with a 'medical model'. In this, it is argued that psychological distress is best understood by reference to the traditional medical concepts such as aetiology, diagnosis, prognosis, etc. Psychiatric problems are given disease names and discussed under the heading 'psychopathology'. This model endorses the two basic tenets of positivism mentioned above; thus it is assumed that it is possible and preferable to make observations objectively in psychiatry. Just as physical medicine characterizes a patient's condition in terms of temperature, pulse, blood pressure and other measurable phenomena so too psychiatry attempts to measure the 'symptoms' of psychological distress in an objective manner. To this end, various 'instruments' have been developed. These take the form of standardized questionnaires, which seek to identify and quantify psychiatric disorders in a precise and replicable fashion. Great effort has also been put into the development of operational definitions of symptoms and syndromes culminating in the now widely used *Diagnostic and Statistical Manual* of the American Psychiatric Association.

Psychiatry has also sought to produce theoretical models based upon causal modes of explanation. As David Ingleby has shown, this has taken both 'strong' and 'weak' forms:

> The 'strong' form, variously called the 'faulty-machine' or 'disease' model, suggests that the causal factors underlying mental illness are physiological disorders; the 'weak' version still invokes causal explanation, but blames the problems on psychological or environmental factors.
>
> (Ingleby 1980: 34)

Ingleby argues that the positivist position is not eliminated by simply denying the physiological origins of madness and distress and arguing instead for an alternative set of aetiological factors (whether these be psychological or social). Both forms of this theoretical model assume that psychiatric problems can be explained by analysing the effects of various 'causal' factors. This is an important point because many critics of psychiatry have specifically targeted the medical model, or the 'strong' positivist position, arguing that psychiatry's problems are all due to the stranglehold of the medical profession.[10]

Two important consequences which result from psychiatry's adoption of the positivist position in both its medical and non-medical forms are, first, the conclusion that psychological problems have the same basic form cross-culturally and, second, that the history of psychiatry can be seen as a progressive identification of the true nature of mental illness. Through the adoption of the 'scientific method' and the use of standardized questionnaires and operational criteria, psychiatric research has attempted to delineate the universal aspects of mental illnesses. Because such questionnaires and criteria are produced within the context of a positivist science, they are thought of as value-free and 'neutral'. They are not felt to incorporate any particular ethnic or social class bias. Their use in non-Western societies is seen as unproblematic and the results produced are seen as universally valid. The fundamental assumption is that there is equivalence between human thoughts, emotions and behaviours on the one side and objects of the natural world such as rocks, plants, livers and brains on the other. Just as the latter have the same form regardless of history or geography, it is assumed that the phenomena of human life are similarly open to objective description.

On the other hand positivism underscores psychiatry's claim to be in the process of unravelling the true nature of mental illness. As I have noted above, inherent in the positivist position is the assumption that science is a progressive endeavour. It is seen as leading inexorably towards a deeper understanding of how the world, including human beings, functions. Scientific psychiatry holds that it, too, is leading to a deeper and continually more accurate picture of the nature of mental illness. Sir Martin Roth, founding President of Britain's Royal College of Psychiatrists, in a book written with Jerome Kroll, asserts that:

> . . . having regard to the successes of the medical models in recent decades, we can reasonably expect that clinical practice and the public health approaches to the problems of mental health will acquire a more solid factual foundation and thus become more precise and effective. This is because medical models pose clear questions that can be refuted or upheld by scientific investigation.
>
> (Roth and Kroll 1986: 66)

This sort of position fits happily with an account of psychiatry's history that emphasizes its progressive nature. In such an account it is proposed that in the modern Western world we are enjoying the fruits of a scientific enlightenment which has allowed us to discover that psychiatric problems are not due to witchcraft, possession or any other supernatural force but are the effects of disease processes, whether organic or psychological. We look back on centuries of barbarism when the mentally sick were not treated properly. As Peter Sedgwick puts it:

> The basic perspective of this variety of psychiatric history is, roughly speaking, liberal, evolutionist and sympathetic to modern diagnostic categories as the criterion of reality against which earlier discoveries are to be tested and found wanting.
>
> (Sedgwick 1982: 129)

In the positivist account, madness is seen to be waiting for psychiatry to describe and classify it. From this position, the object of a science is seen to exist prior to the science, which slowly begins to apprehend and eventually understand it. Knowledge is seen to develop in an evolutionary and teleological fashion. This position has been challenged recently from a number of directions. I will not discuss these critiques here. My aim has been simply to highlight the relationship between psychiatry and the cultural agenda initiated by the European Enlightenment. However, as I will return to the work of Michel Foucault later in this work, I would like to briefly mention his work in this area. The positivist account of the history of psychiatry is one that Foucault opposed strenuously. Instead, he argued that madness could not have become the object of a special science, as it did to psychiatry in the nineteenth century, unless it was previously the object of exclusion, internment and correction. Alan Sheridan summarizes Foucault's position thus:

> Madness did not wait, in immobile identity, for the advent of psychiatry to carry it from the darkness of superstition to the light of truth. The categories of modern psychiatry were not lying in a state of nature waiting to be picked up by the perceptive observer: they were produced by that 'science' in its very act of formation. Similarly, the sudden, massive resort to confinement in the mid-seventeenth century was not a necessary response to a sudden upsurge of 'asocial elements'. This act was as sudden as that by which the lepers were expelled from the city: but its significance cannot be reduced to its actual result.
>
> (Sheridan 1980: 26)

I ask the reader to keep this tension in mind when while we examine the question of trauma and meaning and how psychiatry has sought to explore both.

II Cognitivism and the question of meaning

So far in this chapter I have argued that one result of the European Enlightenment has been a cultural preoccupation with reason and rationality. This was evident in the philosophy of Descartes, which, as we have seen above, is still influential in psychology and psychiatry. Another important product of the Enlightenment is the dominance of a positivist paradigm within psychiatry. In essence, positivism asserts the possibility of framing all human problems in a technical idiom. It is proposed that such problems can be investigated adequately with the tools of a causal science and solutions developed accordingly. While commentators such as Bolton and Hill argue that biological and psychological sciences require a concept of 'intentional causality' they remain broadly committed to the positivist agenda.

In the rest of this chapter I shall examine the growing importance of cognitivism in psychology and psychiatry and indicate how this process has been supported by (and in turn has offered support to) what is known as a functionalist approach within philosophy of mind. As shall become clear, functionalism is premised upon both the rationalist and empiricist principles of what I have called Cartesianism and sought to outline above.

The growing popularity of cognitivism

For most readers, cognitivism is perhaps best introduced through a discussion of its use in clinical situations. In recent years cognitive therapy has become very popular in psychiatry and psychology and some variant of it is now prescribed regularly for a range of psychiatric problems including anxiety, depression, symptoms of psychosis as well as post-traumatic conditions. It is a form of therapy that appears 'clear' in its concepts and is relatively easy to learn. It also appears able to define its operations and to measure and quantify its benefits. Its popularity is understandable in the midst of a culture that places a high priority on efficiency. However, as we shall see, cognitive therapy, like all other forms of psychotherapy, is based on a certain set of assumptions concerning the nature of the self and its relationships to others and to the world in general. In fact, the therapeutic element is just one aspect of an overall approach to psychology. It is premised upon the 'cognitive model' of mind, in which disorders of mind are understood to be caused by 'dysfunctional beliefs' and 'faulty information processing'. Cognitivism has become popular, not only in the area of therapy, but as we shall see below, across most of the sub-disciplines of psychology.

The cognitivist approach to 'mind' and its disorders

Cognitivism is essentially a paradigm, a framework, through which researchers have found an order in human reality and a way to explore this reality. Within any paradigm there are competing theories and approaches. I will not attempt to give a comprehensive overview of all the different approaches that could be called cognitivist. I will attempt to give a general description of cognitivism which I believe accurately reflects the model at work in most psychiatric research. This account is broadly based on Rom Harré's and Grant Gillett's characterization of cognitivism in their book *The Discursive Mind* (1994). This refers to a cognitivism that involves a computational approach to thought. While this has been challenged by approaches that rely on connectionist models, computational approaches are still central in cognitivist accounts of trauma (see below).

The basic premise of cognitivism is that there is an underlying structure to mentation. This structure is based on the biological organi-zation of the brain but needs a separate, non-biological, set of concepts to fully grasp it. In this model the brain is akin to computer hardware, whereas the mind, or mental activity, is like the software: the programmes that run on the basis of the hardware. In this framework it is logical to treat the brain and the mind as separate realms and the project of cognitivism is about exploring the structures and the underlying basic elements of the software, of the mind. While the content of these programmes might differ between cultural groups the form of the programmes remains the same. Because of this, cognitivism involves an adherence to the positivist agenda of exploring the mind through the framework of causal science. It also involves adherence to a model of psychological universalism, in which thought and emotion are understood to involve similar basic elements and structures cross-culturally. The challenge for cognitivism is to delineate the nature of these underlying structures and to allow for therapeutic developments based on this understanding.

While cognitivism retains the same positivist scientific approach that guided behaviourism, it has wanted to explore the contents of the 'black box' which lies between stimulus and response. As Harré and Gillett put it:

> Cognitive psychologists attempted to understand the mechanisms that mediated the transition from stimulus to response by examining such things as semantic categorization and its effect on recall of information, explicit instructions and problem-solving strategies, the effect of cognitive anticipations on perception, the relationship between images and propositions in the internal processes subserving cognition, the hierarchical relationships between categories in the ordering and retrieval of knowledge. The overall model was that the mind was an internal realm of operations and computations hypotheses that could be tested by experimental tests of their logical consequences via the systematic manipulation of specifiable inputs and outputs to the black box of cognition.
>
> (Harré and Gillett 1994: 15)

A fundamental assumption is that these mechanisms can be characterized in causal terms and thus causal hypotheses generated which can then be used to produce predictions of what behaviour will be produced under certain sets of circumstances:

> In the conception of the information processing model, it seemed that psychology had now found a format that would allow it to become fully scientific, in the realist sense. Its theories would consist of hypotheses about information processing mechanisms. Predictions, describing behaviour, could be drawn from these hypotheses. All forms of activity including the use of speech, the display of emotions, the evincing of attitudes, the solving of problems, and so on ought to be comprehensible in principle.
>
> (Harré and Gillett 1994: 14)

As cognitivism has become increasingly influential, more and more areas of psychology have come to adopt the paradigm. Thus in developmental psychology, under the influence of Piaget, there has been a preoccupation with the kinds of operations that can be performed by a developing subject at different stages, and with the underlying structures which underpin these. In personality theory there has been a shift towards an examination of the cognitive framework of the subject. Personal Construct

Theory emerged in the 1960s and has become increasingly popular as formulations based on unconscious drives and traits have faded (Kelly 1955). The idea that human beings operate personally and socially on the basis of unconscious models and rules has become something of an orthodoxy. These models and rules have been formulated differently, and the terminology has also differed, but the basic proposition has remained the same. Thus there are the 'rules and roles' described by Rom Harré in an early model of social behaviour (Harré and Secord 1973). There are also the concepts of internal, cognitive 'scripts' described by Schank and Abelson (1977), and the 'grammars' of linguists influenced by Chomsky. The concept of unconscious 'schemas' is currently very popular. The social psychologist Ronnie Janoff-Bulman defines the term in the following quotations:

> Yet, in all instances, whether the organized knowledge is about a common object or a broad class of people, the relevant schema is essentially a theory that goes beyond the data given. A schema is not simply a straightforward accumulation of specific original instances and encounters but rather a generalization or abstraction involving organized knowledge about a stimulus or concept.

> Our fundamental assumptions about the world are essentially our grandest schemas, our most abstract, generalized knowledge structures.

> Schema research demonstrates the theory-driven (rather than data-driven) nature of our perceptual and cognitive processes.
>
> (Janoff-Bulman 1992: 29)

She quotes Daniel Goleman:

> . . . schemas embody the rules and categories that order raw experience into coherent meaning. All knowledge and experience is packaged in schemas. Schemas are the ghost in the machine, the intelligence that guides information as it flows through the mind.
>
> (Goleman 1985: 75)

In clinical psychiatry the notion that human beings operate with unconscious models or schemas has been used in a number of ways. We shall see in the next chapter how this approach has become dominant in the area of post-traumatic conditions. However, it was in relation to the clinical syndrome of depression that cognitive therapy first achieved prominence. Indeed, Aaron Beck's theory of depression has become something of an 'exemplar' in psychiatry and has guided thinking in many other areas.

Beck proposed that in the person who later develops depression, faulty or dysfunctional assumptions are laid down as cognitive schemas in early life. They are activated by critical incidents in later life and a meshing between the particular incident and the dysfunctional assumptions brings about a complex of 'negative automatic thoughts'. These thoughts underlie the clinical state of depression and are essentially distorted, negative, dysfunctional and unhelpful. He says:

> In brief, the theory postulates that the depressed or depression-prone individual has certain idiosyncratic patterns (schemas) which may become activated whether by specific stresses impinging on specific vulnerabilities, or by overwhelming non-specific stresses. When the cognitive patterns are activated, they tend to dominate the individual's thinking and to produce the affective and motivational phenomena associated with depression.
>
> (Beck 1972: 129–30)

Depression is, for Beck, not simply an affective (or mood) disturbance but rather involves a specific disorder of thinking, of cognition. In contrast to the disorder of thought characteristically seen in conditions labelled schizophrenic, depression does not involve a disorder of rationality as such:

> . . . the ideas are generally not irrational, but are too absolute, broad and extreme; too highly personalized; and are used too arbitrarily to help the patient to handle the exigencies of his life.
>
> (Beck 1976: 246)

The 'cognitive disorder' involved in depression can be defined in terms of: overgeneralization, selective abstraction and negativism. For Beck, depression is a specific condition with a specific form of psychopathology and a specific form of therapy to match. It involves the patient's cognitions being out of step with the surrounding culture in a specific way, a distorted way that requires a specific form of therapeutic intervention. In contrast to dynamic approaches, cognitive therapy does not involve any great exploration of the past. It is very much focused on the 'here and now'. It does not theorize about the relationship between patient and therapist in terms of unconscious forces, or in terms of transference and counter-transference. It involves the therapist in 'training' the patient to examine his/her thoughts in a systematic and 'non-distorted' way. The patient, in turn, is involved in 'homework' and 'exercises' which are carried out between sessions. The therapist's job is basically to help the patient confront his/her cognitive distortions, and, largely through blunt persuasion, provide much of the motivation for the patient to carry out the homework.

The emergence of cognitivism

There are many reasons for the emergence of the 'first cognitive revolution' in psychology (Harré and Gillett 1994). Clinical and theoretical psychology had limited scope to develop within the strict confines of a behavioural paradigm. Behavioural approaches in psychology and psychotherapy were in many ways the direct legacy of the empiricist tradition in science. Behaviourism involved a relegation of mental processes, including reason, to a minor role in influencing human action. As Kenneth Gergen puts it:

> In many respects, the behaviourist and neo-behaviourist movements in psychology recapitulate, at the theoretical level, the empiricist emphasis in the philosophy of science. That is, the theories of human psychology represent reformulations of the empiricist metatheory that informs the behaviourist and neo-behaviourist projects of science . . . However, these movements simultaneously left unexplored the rationalist contribution to the reigning metatheory. Unexplored was the implicit implicature, in which rationalist processes could be credited with a contribution to human action – not simply pawns to antecedent conditions, but possessing intrinsic properties with their own demands on action.
>
> (Gergen 1995: 13–14)

Behavioural approaches refused to engage with the 'inner voice', the internal aspects of mind. The advent of cognitive models and therapies represented a fundamental shift in psychology to an acceptance not only of the mind's existence, but also an acceptance of the central premise of rationalism: the primacy of thought over sensation and the experiential world. In the cognitivist paradigm active mental processes come to have a central and dominant role in directing human action. In putting the emphasis on internal thought and reason and also making this open to scientific observation, it would appear that cognitivism finally brings together the two great Enlightenment traditions we discussed above: rationalism and empiricism.

As well as a growing dissatisfaction with the limitations of strict empiricism and behaviourism, the emergence of the computer as a cultural icon in the West has been an important factor. Computer language is now part of the vernacular in many parts of the world. Computer images and metaphors inform many discussions about ourselves and our activities. In the past 20 years it has become possible not only to think of the mind as being *like* a computer, but also to propose that the mind *is* a computer. As psychology became concerned to understand the mind in terms of causal mechanisms and various versions of rule-following formulae it found a natural ally in the developing world of artificial intelligence (AI). In fact the assumptions underlying AI and cognitivist psychology are essentially the same. If it is possible, in principle, to account for different aspects of human thought and behaviour in terms of rule-following formulae, then, also in principle, it should be possible to build machines which would operate on the basis of these formulae and so replicate human intelligence and behaviour. Both developments assume that the human mind works in the same way that computers do. Two major early proponents of AI, Newell and Simon, conclude that their work:

> ... provide(s) a general framework for understanding problem-solving behaviour ... and finally reveals with great clarity that free behaviour of a reasonably intelligent human can be understood as the product of a complex but finite and determinate set of laws.
>
> (Newell and Simon 1963: 293)

Philosophical assumptions of the cognitivist paradigm

I have already argued that cognitivism is, in essence, a modern-day version of Cartesianism. I defined the latter in terms of methodological individualism, separation of 'inner' mind from 'outer' body and surrounding world, and a positivist causal understanding of human reality. In this section I will develop this argument further.

Functionalism

Theoretical and practical developments in AI and in cognitive psychology have been given substantial support from contemporary developments in philosophy of mind. Philosophers such as Jerry Fodor argue the case for a computational view of thought, a position that is perhaps the dominant one in current philosophy of mind (Crane 1995). Functionalism, as this philosophy of mind has come to be called, has, in fact, become 'something approaching an orthodoxy over the last ten years' (Lyons 1995: lviii).

Functionalism involves the belief that mental states are defined by their causes and effects. It asserts a distinction between *role* and *occupant*. Thus a similar functional state can be *realized* in different systems. In many ways a response to, and a rejection of, the ideas of eliminative materialism[11], functionalists draw on the dualism implicit in the computer model to argue the case for a separate mental realm. Just as computer software cannot be fully accounted for by reference to hardware alone, so too mental states cannot be reductively explained through an account of brain states alone. Mentation has its own elements and structures, which cannot be explained in the language of physics, chemistry and neurophysiology. There are, now, a number of separate versions of functionalism. In his book *Mind, Language and Reality*, Hilary Putnam made the case for 'computer functionalism' (also called 'Turing machine functionalism'):

> According to functionalism, the behaviour of, say, a computing machine
> is not explained by the physics and chemistry of the computing
> machine. It is explained by the machine's *program*. Of course, that
> program is realized in a particular physics and chemistry, and could,
> perhaps, be deduced from that physics and chemistry. But that does not
> make the program a physical or chemical property of the machine: it is
> an abstract property of the machine. Similarly, I believe that the psycho-
> logical properties of human beings are not physical and chemical
> properties of human beings, although they may be realized by physical
> and chemical properties of human beings.
>
>   (Putnam 1975: xiii)

The mind is not only separable from the body (brain) in functionalist
accounts but also from the world around. It is a realm which exists in
relation to this outside world and which represents it. Mental operations
exist in a self-contained internal domain. Thus while functionalists reject
(Cartesian) ontological dualism they continue to think (in a Cartesian
idiom) about the mind as something 'interior' and separable from an
'external' world. This echoes my discussion of Bolton and Hill in Part I of
this chapter.

   In addition to its assertion of the mind-brain distinction, functionalism also makes assertions about the nature of thinking. It proposes that
representational mental states, such as beliefs, desires, memories, and
aspirations are related to one another in a computational way. They are
processed in a rule-governed way, as are the representational states of a
computer. Fodor calls this the 'Representational Theory of Mind'. He
writes:

> At the heart of this theory is the postulation of a language of thought: an
> infinite set of 'mental representations' which function both as the
> immediate objects of propositional attitudes and as the domains of
> mental processes.

Fodor spells out what the notion of 'propositional attitude' means for
him:

> To believe that such and such is to have a mental symbol that means
> such and such tokened in your head in a certain way; it's to have such a
> token 'in your belief box' . . . Correspondingly, to hope that such and
> such is to have a token of that same mental symbol tokened in your
> head, but in a different way; it's to have it tokened 'in your hope box'.

Furthermore, this theory of mind involves the claim that:

> Mental processes are causal sequences of tokenings of mental represen-
> tations.
>
> (Fodor 1995: 258)

Thus functionalism, as a theory of mind, incorporates assumptions that emerge from the Cartesian tradition, discussed above. Its focus is the individual 'mind', which is understood to be 'something' which exists in relation to an 'outside' world. The contents of the mental realm are held to exist in 'causal' relations with each other, and are thus open to scientific investigation.

We shall see in Section II how a Heideggerian perspective challenges the basic tenets of Cartesianism and puts these assumptions in question. However, before outlining such a Heideggerian perspective it is first important to identify a further assumption that also underscores current cognitivist approaches in psychology. This involves a particular orientation to the question of time, in particular, to how past and present are related.

Time and causality in the cognitivist framework

Within functionalism, meaningful behaviour is understood to be an outcome of intentional mental states, which can be characterized in terms of representations. In this framework the meaning of a piece of behaviour consists of those mental representations in the mind of the person involved which give rise to the behaviour. Grasping the meaning of a piece of text involves correctly accounting for the system of representations in the mind of the author. Because all mental states are held to be represen-tational, in this framework there is, in principle at least, a single correct answer to the question of what the meaning of any piece of behaviour is. It is always theoretically possible to provide a full account of the system of representations in a person's mind at any given time. Cognitivism is concerned with how these representations are structured and related to one another. As Jerome Wakefield puts it:

> The cognitivist holds that representational states are determinate in
> meaning because the content of a mental sentence or a mental picture,
> like the contents of sentences and pictures generally, can be discerned
> and described from their structure alone. If meanings are inherently
> determinate, then an interpretation is an attempt to use language to
> match as closely as possible the actual content of the intentional state,
> and the interpretation either gets it exactly right or suffers from some
> degree of inexactitude.
>
> (Wakefield 1988: 135)

In the cognitivist view the relationship between past and present involves a relationship between such determinate intentional states. Furthermore, the move from one intentional state to another comes about through interactions with the external world, which can be characterized in terms of operations and thus systematically defined. Just as the software in a computer can be changed by inputs from a keyboard, so too schemas in the human mind can be changed through inputs from the experiences of the individual. Within cognitivism, memory plays an extremely important role. It is the matrix in which past and present are related. Memory is essentially about storage and retrieval and again computer models have helped organize theoretical developments in this area. In this framework past and present are clearly separable states of mind. The model of time that underlines this framework involves a linear series of 'nows'. For the human being each 'now' involves a particular intentional state of mind, with certain representations organized in a particular way. Just as the contents of any particular mental state can be defined and formalized, so too change from one state to another can be accounted for in terms of certain causal laws. These laws are themselves fixed and atemporal. Memory involves reaching out of the present. As Frederick Olafson says:

> . . . memory is typically construed in terms of episodic acts in the course of which we reach out of the present and back into the past so as to recapture something from our earlier life. The facts that are so recovered may also be thought of as having been 'stored' after their actuality had lapsed and, as so stored, continuing on with us through each of the successive presents in which we live.
>
> (Olafson 1987: 86)

In the next chapter we shall see how post-traumatic sequelae are understood to be the result of a disordered interaction of past and present conceived in causal terms. In Section II we shall see how Heideggerian phenomenology offers a very different approach to the question of time and causality.

Summary

In this chapter I have argued that psychiatry is very much a product of the European Enlightenment and its concern with reason and interiority. In many ways, cognitivist psychology has involved a certain crystallization of these concerns. Cognitivism is about an ordering of mind in a way that makes it amenable to scientific investigation; it incorporates a marriage of rationalism and empiricism. Cognitive approaches have come to occupy a central space in both psychiatry and psychology and cognitive therapy is moving to replace psychoanalysis in the world of psychotherapy. I have shown how this approach incorporates the basic assumptions of

Cartesianism. Specifically it incorporates an individualist and positivist approach to the understanding of human reality. It works with the basic assumption that the mind exists as separate from, and in relation to, an outside world. This tradition informs much of what might be called 'common-sense' ideas about the self and the nature of thought in much of modern Western society. Cognitivism understands the meaningfulness of the world as something internal, something generated by the interaction of our schemas with sensory data and other inputs. It is something that can be researched and analysed with the tools of scientific positivism. Cognitivism also operates with a linear model of time and causality. In the next chapter I shall examine how this works in regard to the issue of trauma.

One of the central arguments developed in this book is the need for an approach to human reality which pays due regard to importance of context. In other words, I am attempting to approach the questions of meaning and trauma from a perspective which avoids a commitment to a strong notion of 'interior' mind. I shall look to continental philosophy to ground this endeavour and in particular to the work of Heidegger. However, I am aware that Heidegger's phenomenology is only one of a number of approaches that involve a critique of Cartesianism and attempt to get beyond it. A number of Wittgenstein-inspired philosophers have developed *externalist* accounts of mind. For example, this is the position put forward by Gregory McCulloch (1995) in his book *The Mind and its World*. Perhaps the most influential move in this direction is that developed in the most recent work of Hilary Putnam. In *Representation and Reality* (1988) Putnam argues against his original functionalist position (see above) and what he calls 'mentalism'. Button et al. (1995) draw on the work of both Wittgenstein and Gilbert Ryle in their critique of cognitivism and functionalism. I will mention Wittgenstein in a number of places in the text but there is no systematic development of his ideas in this work.

I have also avoided any real encounter with the world of 'connectionism'. When I write about cognitivism, I have in mind approaches in psychology which look to traditional computer-based models of information processing. I avoid connectionism because it has not, as yet, had any great influence on theoretical approaches to meaning, trauma and PTSD.[12] Theories of PTSD are currently dominated by concerns with 'schemas', 'appraisal mechanisms', 'event cognitions' and other concepts, which draw heavily on the assumptions of computational approaches to mind and thought. There is considerable debate at present about the implications of connectionist (or neural network) models for work in psychology and philosophy. Some commentators argue that these models do not substantially challenge the traditional cognitivist paradigm.[13] However, others argue that connectionism involves a radical new paradigm, which has major philosophical implications. The latter view is developed by Paul Cilliers in his book *Complexity and Postmodernism: Understanding Complex Systems* (1998). Cilliers suggests that connectionism moves us away from cognitivism's traditional philosophical dependence on analytical philosophy and points, instead, to its compatibility with post-structuralist philosophies. He remarks that it is strange that:

> . . . when it comes to descriptions of the functioning of the brain, an obviously relational structure, there is still such a strong adherence to atomic representation and deterministic algorithms. One of the reasons for this must surely be that cognitive science inherited its methodological framework from a deterministic, analytical tradition. Post-structural theory, I claim, assists us in revising this position.
>
> (Cilliers 1998: 35)

If Cilliers is correct, then it is possible that (in the future) connectionism will serve as a bridge between the sort of context-centred approach to psychology developed in this work and the world of neuroscience.

Chapter 3
Post-traumatic anxiety

Introduction

In 1980, the American Psychiatric Association included the diagnosis 'Post Traumatic Stress Disorder' in the third edition of its Diagnostic and Statistical Manual, the so-called *DSM III* (APA 1980). The inclusion of Post Traumatic Stress Disorder (PTSD) not only reflected an increasing interest in the area of trauma on the part of psychiatrists and psychologists, but also in itself provided a spur to further research and the development of ideas in this area. Within the past 15 years the concept has been taken up widely in North America, Europe and in many other parts of the world. Psychological trauma has become a central preoccupation of psychiatry during this period. Blake et al. (1992) have documented the striking increase in published work on trauma in the years between 1970 and 1989. Many special clinics have opened for the treatment of post-traumatic disorders; there are now several international journals dedicated to the subject and new books appear almost weekly, covering different aspects of trauma and its sequelae. The editors of a recent volume declared that PTSD is the 'diagnosis of the 1990s' (Marsella et al. 1996a).

Prior to the inclusion of PTSD in the *DSM III* of 1980, psychiatry had made a clear separation between the acute reaction to stress and more enduring consequences. For example, in *DSM I* (APA 1952) the entity 'gross stress reaction' was conceived as a disorder which resolved rapidly unless there was pre-existing personality pathology. Similarly, *DSM II* (APA 1968) included the disorder 'transient situational disturbance' which was said to be present if the response to a stressful event was short-lived. If more long-lasting effects were noted then the disorder became simply 'anxiety neurosis'. Again, this implied that stress responses were short-lived unless the individual patient had some pre-existing vulnerability. *DSM II* is quite clear about this: 'if the patient has good adaptive capacity his symptoms usually recede as the stress diminishes. If, however, the

45

symptoms persist after the stress is removed, the diagnosis of another mental disorder is indicated'.

Thus *DSM III* PTSD represents a considerable shift, in that it involves the notion that traumatic events in adulthood can, of themselves, produce prolonged adverse psychological consequences. There is a moral implication to this change. If trauma can, of itself, produce prolonged psychiatric sequelae, then responsibility for this suffering lies outside the patient, with whoever or whatever caused the trauma. On the other hand if prolonged morbidity only occurs in someone with pre-existing problems, then this responsibility is somewhat lessened. Allan Young (1995) argues that this moral issue was one of the main reasons why PTSD achieved full nosological status in the USA classification in 1980, at the end of the war in Vietnam. Young cites the work of Wilbur Scott, who interviewed the principal people involved in getting PTSD recognized. Scott points out that during the 1970s American psychiatrists and other mental health professionals, particularly those working in the Veterans Administration (VA) medical system, were faced with a virtual epidemic of suicides and severe psychiatric problems among veterans returned from Vietnam. A number of veterans and their supporters started to become frustrated with a psychiatric system which attached little importance to their terrible experiences during the war:

> Mental health professionals across the country assessed disturbed Vietnam veterans using diagnostic nomenclature that contained no specific entries for war-related trauma . . . VA physicians typically did not collect military histories as part of their diagnostic work-up. Many thought Vietnam veterans who were agitated by their war experiences, or who talked repeatedly about them, suffered from a neurosis or psychosis whose origin and dynamics lay outside the realm of combat.
>
> (Scott 1990: 298)

Gradually a campaign emerged involving veterans, their families, politicians and prominent psychiatric clinicians. This aimed at achieving full official recognition of the role of wartime suffering in the causation of psychopathology. As Young notes:

> . . . the advocates were able to make a compelling *moral* argument for PTSD, albeit one that fell on deaf ears in the VA and the traditional veterans' organizations. The failure to make a place for PTSD would be equivalent to blaming the victim for his misfortunes – misfortunes inflicted on him by both his government and its enemies. It would mean denying medical care and compensation to men who had been obliged or induced to sacrifice their youths in a dirty and meaningless war. Acknowledging PTSD would be a small step toward repaying a debt.
>
> (Young 1995: 114)

Contrary to the dominant positivist perspective (as outlined in the last chapter), Young argues that PTSD was *created* at a particular time, in a particular place and according to a particular moral and political agenda. It was not simply a medical condition waiting to be discovered. It fulfilled the need of American society to recognize the suffering of the young people who were damaged by the war in Vietnam. This is not, of course, how psychiatry sees it. As Scott (1990) notes, those psychiatrists and others involved in the campaign for the recognition of PTSD saw it as an 'always-already-there object in the world'. It was understood to be a hidden and neglected syndrome, and they were fighting for its 'recognition'. Interestingly, at the same time that PTSD was being 'recognized', homosexuality was being 'de-recognized' as a psychiatric condition that did not appear in the *DSM III*.

However, the *DSM* claims to be 'a-theoretical' and based purely on scientific investigation. As a result, this background agenda is given little attention in psychiatric discussions of trauma. PTSD is presented as a 'straightforward' medical condition, which can be defined in terms of aetiology, diagnosis, psychopathology, treatment and prognosis. The 'symptoms' described in the *DSM* are held to be universal and not associated with any particular cultural situation.

In this chapter I will first describe the 'syndrome' of PTSD as presented in the *DSM*. I will then examine theoretical approaches to PTSD and show how cognitivism has come to be of central importance in current understandings of the syndrome. In the next chapter I shall examine a literature that challenges the universality of PTSD and calls into question some of the underlying assumptions built into the concept.

The syndrome of post-traumatic stress disorder

According to the recent versions of the American Psychiatric Association's *DSM* a diagnosis of PTSD can be made if the patient exhibits a certain combination of symptoms. These symptoms fall into three groups:

1. Symptoms of intrusion; such as recurrent thoughts about the trauma, nightmares, flashbacks and exaggerated reactions upon exposure to reminders of the trauma. These are also known as 're-experiencing' symptoms.
2. Symptoms of constriction and avoidance; such as efforts to avoid thoughts about the trauma, efforts to avoid places or activities that remind one of the trauma and evidence of more general withdrawal from the world.
3. Other symptoms such as irritability, insomnia, poor concentration and hypervigilance. These 'other' symptoms are sometimes described as 'hyperarousal symptoms'.

In the 1980 *DSM III* the last group of symptoms included feelings of guilt about surviving when others had not and the presence of an exaggerated startle response. This version also described three forms of PTSD: acute, when the onset of symptoms was within six months of the trauma and the duration was less than six months; chronic, when the duration was for more than six months; and delayed, when the symptoms were not present in the first six months after the trauma. The *DSM III* was quite clear that the symptoms were the direct result of the trauma, even though there was an acknowledgement that pre-trauma psychopathology could be a predisposing factor.

In 1987, a revised version of the Diagnostic and Statistical Manual was produced: *DSM III-R* (APA 1987). In this, the third group of symptoms were named as symptoms of 'increased arousal' and survivor guilt was dropped from the criteria. *DSM III-R* had an expanded list of avoidance symptoms. It also asserted that symptoms must usually begin in the immediate aftermath of the trauma and last for no less than one month. In addition, the revised version elaborated an account of the syndrome in children. Like the original *DSM III* it continued the idea that the traumatic event was the central aetiological factor.

By the time the next version was produced in 1994, psychiatric thinking about the syndrome had shifted somewhat and a number of important alterations were made. In the *DSM IV* (APA 1994) account of PTSD a stronger role is given to individual history and personality. The new version also incorporates recent thinking about the stressor criterion. Thus, it is acknowledged that being a *witness* to a distressing event can be traumatizing, even in the absence of direct threat to self. While in *DSM III* the stressor criterion simply reads:

> The existence of a recognizable stressor that would evoke significant symptoms of distress in almost anyone,

in *DSM IV* this has changed to:

> The person has been exposed to a traumatic event in which both the following were present:
> (1) The person experienced, witnessed, or was confronted with an event or events that involved actual or threatened death or serious injury, or a threat to the physical integrity of self or others.
> (2) The person's response involved fear, helplessness, or horror. *Note*: In children, this may be expressed instead by disorganized or agitated behaviour.

DSM IV also included a new category: Acute Stress Disorder. This is separate from PTSD and to make the diagnosis the symptoms must occur within four weeks of the trauma and resolve within that four-week period. In spite of these changes, the characteristic symptoms of PTSD are now widely accepted as defining the essential elements of human reactions to trauma. Within the discourse on trauma there is continuing debate about specific symptoms, and the *DSM* description of PTSD will no doubt continue to be revised. However, there appears to be a consensus about the formulation of post-traumatic reactions in terms of intrusive, constrictive and hyperarousal symptoms. These symptoms are held to be universal and it is argued that they can be seen in children as well as adults. It is assumed that they are expressive of conflicts and disturbances happening within individual minds. As we shall see in the next chapter there is considerable debate about the universal significance of the intrusion/avoidance symptom complex. However, for now I shall assume that these symptoms do occur after the experience of traumatic events. In the rest of this chapter I shall look at how different theoretical approaches have been explored in an effort to understand how and why these symptom patterns emerge. I will not explore the biological literature on PTSD in any depth, apart from a brief look at some interesting neuroendocrinological findings in the next chapter. The biological focus has been primarily upon the hyperarousal symptoms seen in PTSD. Van der Kolk (1996) provides a useful summary of this literature.

Behavioural approaches to PTSD

A number of PTSD researchers have argued that traditional behavioural frameworks are adequate to conceptualize the way in which the clinical syndrome is produced. These involve learning theory and models based on the notion of conditioning. Such researchers point to the similarity between the symptomatology of simple phobias and that of PTSD. In the former there is a recognizable stimulus (trauma), following which the individual shows fear and avoidance when confronted with similar or associated stimuli. In Watson and Rayner's paradigmatic experiment, 'Little Albert' was exposed to a loud and frightening noise when playing with a white rat. Two-year-old Albert subsequently showed fear when exposed to the rat, even when the noise was not present. However, individuals with the syndrome of PTSD fear and 'avoid' a range of situations not directly related to the original fearful situation. This feature needs to be explained by any theory which claims to provide an adequate conceptualization. With this in mind behaviourists have looked to Mowrer's (1960) 'two-factor' learning theory. According to this, two types of learning, classical and instrumental, occur in syndromes involving sustained reactions of fear and avoidance:

In the first stage, via temporal contiguity, a previously neutral stimulus becomes associated with an unconditioned stimulus (UCS) that innately evokes discomfort or fear. The neutral stimulus then acquires aversive properties such that its presence elicits anxiety; it now becomes a conditioned stimulus (CS) for fear responses. When this conditioned stimulus is paired with another neutral stimulus, the latter also acquires aversive overtones and its presentation will also evoke anxiety. Through this higher order conditioning, many stimuli, including words, images and thoughts, acquire the capacity to engender anxiety. The number of conditioned stimuli is further increased via a process of stimulus generalization: Stimuli that are similar to the original conditioning stimulus also gain anxiety-eliciting properties. Anxiety or discomfort is experienced as an aversive or unpleasant state. The second stage, then, consists of the development of learned responses, i.e. avoidance or escape responses, which decrease or terminate the discomfort arising from the presence of the conditioned stimuli.

(Foa et al. 1989: 157)

Thus, in the first stage the victim develops fear of various stimuli and tends to avoid these. In the second stage (involving instrumental learning) he/she develops a range of 'escape' and avoidance behaviours, which are selectively reinforced because they reduce exposure to a noxious stimulus.

This theory has been used to understand the symptoms reported by Vietnam veterans (Keane et al. 1985) and victims of rape. With regard to the latter, Becker et al. (1984) have proposed that the assault situation operates as an unconditioned stimulus (UCS), which provokes extreme anxiety and fear. Originally non-threatening aspects of this situation can subsequently operate as conditioned stimuli (CS) and generate anxiety in the victim, on their own. Thus, rape often leads to a fear of sexual activity, a fear of men in general and to other fears associated with the original assault. To avoid discomfort the victim may avoid sexual encounters entirely and actively inhibit sexual feelings in herself. A similar conceptualization is used by Kilpatrick et al. (1985). They point out that thoughts, words and images associated with the original assault situation can come to provoke anxiety, and thus it becomes extremely difficult for the victim to discuss her experience without anxiety. Because of this, victims may find the therapy context extremely stressful. In spite of this, Kilpatrick et al. are confident about the need to face the 'feared object':

Given that the key element in resolution of a phobia is exposure to the feared object, or extinction, avoidance behaviour must be changed if fear responses are to be reduced.

(Kilpatrick et al. 1985: 119)

Although these theories appear able to account for the fear and avoidance often seen after traumatic experiences, they have difficulty explaining why some events result in simple phobic avoidance while others give rise to the additional symptoms of the PTSD syndrome. In particular, behavioural approaches have difficulty accounting for the re-experiencing symptoms which some researchers regard as the cardinal features of the syndrome.[1] The consensus among theorists of PTSD is that learning theory, on its own, simply cannot account for the intrusive-avoidance symptom complex, which is a key element in the syndrome as presented in the *DSM*. As a result, even former proponents of these behavioural approaches have tended to stress the importance of cognitive elements such as 'appraisal' and 'expectancy' in understanding post-traumatic sequelae. In addition, when it comes to treatment, there is an emerging consensus that some form of processing of the traumatic experience needs to take place:

> If PTSD symptoms are the result of inadequate emotional processing, then therapy, aiming at the reduction of these symptoms, can be perceived as facilitating such processing.
>
> (Rothbaum and Foa 1996: 492)

As we shall see below, cognitivism is now the dominant framework used in conceptual work on trauma. Before discussing this work it is important to look at contributions from the psychodynamic point of view.

Psychodynamic contributions

Trauma played a central role in the early theories of Freud. In his work up to 1896 he held that all adult neurosis had its origins in some form of traumatic event. He distinguished between the 'actual neuroses' and the 'psychoneuroses'. The former originated in sexual frustrations encountered in adult life, while the latter were due to sexual traumas experienced in early life (the so-called 'seduction theory'). Most of his attention was directed towards the latter. While obsessional neurosis was the result of 'active seduction', hysteria was brought about by 'passive seduction'. Hence obsessionality was more common in men while hysteria was more common in women. In his early work with Josef Breuer, Freud expressed a great deal of therapeutic optimism with regard to hysteria:

> Each individual hysterical symptom immediately and permanently disappeared when we had succeeded in bringing clearly to light the memory of the event by which it was provoked and in arousing its accompanying affect, and when the patient had described that event in the greatest possible detail and had put the affect into words.
>
> (Breuer and Freud 1955: 6)[2]

As is well known, between 1896 and 1914, Freud abandoned the seduction theory and with it his ideas about the traumatic origins of neurotic symptoms. Actual traumatic events were never to figure very highly again in his work. However, in *Beyond the Pleasure Principle*, published after the First World War, in 1920, he returned to the subject. In this book he proposed a second model of psychic trauma. He suggested that the ego has a 'stimulus barrier' which acts to control the amount of information and energy entering the psychic system. This varies in different people and thus different people respond to the same event in different ways. Freud hypothesized that traumatic neuroses occur when the mind is overwhelmed and overexcited by stimuli from outside. The mental system becomes overloaded. The excessive excitation disorganizes ego functioning and gives rise to the various different post-traumatic sequelae. This flooding of the ego can lead to psychosis but usually a spontaneous process of recovery and reorganization occurs. However, as James Titchener writes:

> The implication of the traumatic or stressful event at unconscious and conscious levels of understanding and the dreaded memory of the moments of fear and helplessness give it a meaning with widespread effects on individual mental life. Resistances against reexperiencing the event vie with intrusive images of it during the daytime and with dreams of it at night. Conflicts over the guilt of surviving when others did not, neurotic and real guilt about responsibility for the traumatic happening, shame of how one behaved under stress, and the overwhelming feeling of helplessness are all aspects of the psychodynamics of the stress response syndrome.
>
> (Titchener 1986: 11–12)

Psychodynamic theorists tend to emphasize the ways in which traumatic experiences resonate with experiences from infancy and childhood. They point to the ways in which traumas can activate conflicts from the past, conflicts around issues such as safety, trust, parental protection, dependency and autonomy. Marmar et al. write:

> Adult trauma may activate specific pre-oedipal or oedipal constellations, particularly those concerning maternal protection and nurturance, control of emotions and bodily functions, and conflicts about potency, rivalry, aggression, and fears of retaliation. The trauma-activated themes are seen as bridges from current concerns to self-representations, representations of other, affect states, and defences arising during early development periods.
>
> (Marmar et al. 1995: 495)

Freud described the phenomenon of 'repetition compulsion', in which the person re-experiences the traumatic event in an effort to gain mastery over it. This was an important precursor for Horowitz's theory of the 'completion tendency' (discussed below), which has played a major role in cognitive theories of PTSD. However, it should be noted that psychoanalysis has actually influenced psychiatry away from a concern with traumatic phenomena during the greatest part of the twentieth century. As Van Velsen notes:

> . . . classical Freudian analytical theory, with its emphasis on drives,
> instincts and regression, meant that for a long time analysts thought that
> it was not the stressor, in particular, that was traumatic but the recrudes-
> cence of a previously repressed infantile conflict.
>
> (Van Velsen 1997: 61)

In more recent times, analysts have again become interested in the phenomenon of trauma and its sequelae. However most have turned away from the classical analytic theory, and towards cognitive ideas, in this process. Horowitz, who has developed the most influential theoretical account of PTSD, is himself an analyst who has turned towards cognitivism. Marmar et al. (1995), quoted above, put forward the conception of traumatic events activating 'earlier mental schemas'. As we shall see below this is very similar to the ways in which explicitly cognitivist approaches describe what happens. Other analysts have also used the notion of 'schema' in their efforts to understand the effects of trauma and, in particular, its effects on the development of transference and counter-transference reactions. Jacob Lindy writes:

> . . . insofar as schemata not only set off specific posttraumatic reactions
> but act as organizers of everyday experience for traumatized individuals,
> the management of traumatic repetitions within the therapeutic context
> – that is, within the transference and counter transference – becomes
> crucial for the entire recovery process.
>
> (Lindy 1996: 526)

Cognitivism and PTSD

The central concern of cognitivist psychology is information processing. As we saw in the last chapter, there is an underlying assumption that the mind–brain relationship is similar to the relationship between computer software and hardware. The mind is like the programmes running in a computer. These mind-programmes are made up of schemes, which structure the individual's orientation to the world and determine the way in which he/she experiences events in the world. Human beings are said to 'process' information about the world just as a software programme processes information and stores it in particular ways. The cognitivist orientation towards trauma involves the idea that there has been a failure in processing. This can happen for a number of reasons; for example, the pre-existing schemata may have been inadequate or the information contained in the traumatic event may be overwhelming. In turn, as we shall see below, therapeutic approaches involve attempts to promote processing of the traumatic material in different ways.

Cognitive appraisal

We have seen above that both traditional behavioural approaches and classical psychodynamic theory have been found inadequate in the face of the PTSD syndrome, as defined in the *DSM*. They have different short-comings but, in essence, neither are able to provide an adequate conceptualization of the sort of psychological sequelae involved in PTSD and, in particular, the persistence of an intrusion-avoidance symptom complex. A number of researchers have argued that an adequate theory has to cover the fact that human beings try to 'make sense' of their environment. The intrusion-avoidance symptoms are understood to result when this fails. Foa et al. (1989) argue that there is a strong case for a theory which invokes 'meaning concepts' when it comes to the full syndrome of PTSD. They argue that strong evidence for this is the fact that perceived threat is a better predictor for the occurrence of PTSD than actual threat.

Cognitive appraisal is theorized as a process through which individuals attach meanings to events. This has been invoked by a number of researchers in relation to trauma. Thus, both Frank and Stewart (1984) and Schepple and Bart (1983), in studies of women who had been raped, showed that victims who were assaulted in situations where they felt safe were more likely to suffer severe reactions compared to those who were attacked in conditions they themselves had thought to be dangerous. These researchers postulated the existence of cognitive schemas that influence the individual's response to trauma and affect their ability to process it successfully. However, there are limits to what the idea of cognitive appraisal can explain. As Lee and Turner remark:

> By placing the emphasis on pre-existing cognitive schemata, the research further sheds light on possible factors that determine why some individuals but not others develop PTSD, and also its severity of presentation. Yet in terms of offering an overall theoretical perspective of PTSD, these approaches lack a convincing means of explaining the core symptoms of PTSD.
>
> (Lee and Turner 1997: 67)

For example, invoking the notion of cognitive appraisal does not help in an explanation of emotional numbing or why some people develop delayed symptoms.

Information-processing

Perhaps the most influential model of post-traumatic stress disorder is the one developed by Mardi Horowitz in California in the late 1970s. It combines both psychodynamic and cognitivist theories. Horowitz proposed in his book *Stress Response Syndromes* (1986) that traumatic experiences disrupt an individual's life by producing a block in cognitive and emotional processing. Horowitz, echoing Freud, assumes the presence of a 'completion tendency' in which the:

> . . . mind continues to process important new information consciously and unconsciously until the situation or the models change and the reality and the schema of that reality reach accord.
>
> (Horowitz 1986: 100)

A traumatic event presents information which conflicts with pre-existing schemas. There is thus an incongruity which gives rise to distress. This provokes a 'stress response', which involves reappraisal of the event and revision of the schemas. If the event is highly traumatic this process is prolonged. However, until such time as the process is complete, the event remains stored in 'active memory'. Horowitz elaborates his theory in terms of 'cognitive processing' and suggests that there are natural and protective limits to the rate of such processing:

> The recurrence of a familiar nonstressful event is likely to be quickly and automatically assimilated. The cognitive processing will be completed, and the information in active memory storage will be rapidly terminated. The information in novel and stressful events, however, cannot be processed rapidly. Thus the point of relative completion is not achieved, and the active memory retention is not terminated, with relevant codings of information remaining in active storage.
>
> Assuming a limited capacity for processing, such codings will remain stored in active memory even when other programs have greater priority in the hierarchy of claims for channels. These actively stored contents, however, will generally be repeatedly represented. Each episode of representation will trigger a resumption of processing. Thus, whenever this set of information achieves a high enough priority, representation and processing will resume. If the contents are interrupted by controls that regulate priorities, they will remain in coded form in active memory.
>
> (Horowitz 1986: 95)

Because the representation of the traumatic event is stored in active memory it is replayed over and over again, each time causing distress for the individual. To prevent emotional exhaustion, inhibition and facilitation processes become involved and these act as a feedback system which modulates the flow of information. Horowitz argues that the response to trauma has a phasic nature and involves periods of active memory alternating with periods of inhibition. These processes are the mind's innate response to stress and occur in all individuals after all stressful events. If there is a failure of inhibition, intrusive symptoms such as nightmares and flashbacks occur. On the other hand, if inhibition is too strong, symptoms of withdrawal and avoidance occur. According to Horowitz, there are substantial individual variations in the ways in which intrusion and avoidance phenomena interact. He focuses on personality structure and gives examples of reactions to stress in people with hysterical, compulsive and narcissistic personalities.

Like other theorists from the cognitivist tradition, Horowitz uses the concept of internal schemas. As noted above, in cognitivist terms, schemas are held to be similar to the programs running on a computer. Such programs encounter new 'information' from a particular perspective and process it in particular ways. This 'information' is then incorporated by the program, which either changes elements of itself in response to the new 'information' or remains the same. Traumatic experience is held to contradict our 'grandest schemata' and overwhelm our ability to process and incorporate new experiences. As the traumatic experience remains unincorporated it continually presents itself to consciousness in the form of intrusive symptoms. As Bolton and Hill formulate it:

> There is in post-traumatic stress reaction a failure to integrate the trauma into the system of belief about the self and reality.
>
> (Bolton and Hill 1996: 359)

Trauma and the 'magic circle': Janoff-Bulman's 'New psychology of trauma'

I have already drawn attention to the fact that many researchers link the symptom complex of intrusion-avoidance to the victim's search for meaning and we have seen above how cognitive theories which aim to grasp this search for meaning have come to dominate current theoretical work on PTSD. A recurrent theme in this context is the idea that extremely frightening events have the effect of shattering the background assumptions of the individual with regard to him/herself and with regard to the order of the outside world. In the cognitive approach the meaningfulness of our lives is dependent on these assumptions. Cognitivism encounters the issue of meaning not as a metaphysical or philosophical problem but as something amenable to empirical investigation.

In her book *Shattered Assumptions: Towards a New Psychology of Trauma* (1992) Ronnie Janoff-Bulman discusses at length the relationship between trauma and loss of meaning. To my mind she provides the best description of what I called the 'magic circle' (see Chapter 1) from the cognitivist side. Following the cognitivist tradition, she accepts that there is a universal and definable structure to human psychology. She argues that at the 'core of our internal worlds' we all have a set of basic assumptions that guide us in our day-to-day thought and actions. She calls these 'our fundamental assumptions'. She argues that, although different psychologists have used different terminology, it is generally accepted within psychology that such a set of assumptions exists in us all:

> Although different terms are used, there is clearly congruence in these descriptions of a single underlying phenomenon. The reference is to a conceptual system, developed over time, that provided us with expectations about the world and ourselves. This conceptual system is best represented by a set of assumptions or internal representations that reflect and guide our interactions in the world and generally enable us to function effectively.
>
> (Janoff-Bulman 1992: 5)

She argues that the core assumptions, which operate universally, concern the nature of the world around us and the value that we attach to ourselves. On the one hand we appear to assume that the world is meaningful and generally benevolent, on the other we assume that we are, ourselves, worthy human beings. The world, in this case, is our own individual world, made up of our environment and our relationships. Although people may not be fully aware of these assumptions she claims that there is empirical evidence that *in fact* most people operate on the basis of some version or another of these. According to Janoff-Bulman there is evidence, for example, that most people are optimistic about their own future, even when they are more generally pessimistic about the world at large. With regard to the orderliness and meaningfulness of the world, she suggests that:

> We generally believe in an action-outcome contingency, that we can control what happens to us, and such a belief provides us with one means of maintaining a view of the world as a meaningful place. In fact, we tend to perceive a contingency between what we do and what happens to us, even in situations when this is clearly inappropriate.
>
> (Janoff-Bulman 1992: 10)

She suggests that a belief in a God who rewards a moral existence also reflects this deeper belief in the orderliness of the world. With regard to the self, Janoff-Bulman maintains that most people evaluate themselves as good and worthy. She says:

> In study after study, people report themselves as better than others and certainly better than average in terms of their own abilities and personal qualities, and scores on self-esteem scales tend to be highly skewed towards the positive end of the scale.
>
> (Janoff-Bulman 1992: 12)

These basic assumptions about ourselves and our worlds are said to be laid down early in life and are generally resistant to change. However, such positive orientations are dependent on an early environment characterized by love and trust. She quotes Eric Erikson's notion of the 'task' of the very first year of life being the establishment of a 'sense of basic trust' in the world. According to Erikson this is dependent on a positive relationship between mother and child. She also quotes the attachment theories of John Bowlby in which children are understood to form 'working models' of the world and themselves through their early relationships with 'attachment figures'.

Janoff-Bulman believes that our assumptions about the world are held in our minds in the form of 'schemas'. Research on schemas tends to show that people are inclined to preserve schemas and do not change them easily. They tend towards 'cognitive conservatism' and, in relation to their mental schemas, are generally resistant to change. Traumatic experiences, however, can have the effect of shattering our deepest schemas, our most fundamental assumptions:

> Over the past fifteen years my students and I have studied a number of victimized populations, including individuals who have experienced rape, battering, and other crimes; life-threatening illnesses, particularly cancer, severe accidents resulting in paralysis; and premature unexpected deaths of parents and spouses. We have attempted to understand the responses of trauma survivors through both intensive interviewing and through quantitative measures of their reactions. For some survivors, the trauma is relatively short-lived, for others it lasts years. Yet regardless of population, and regardless of research approach, we have found remarkable similarities across different victim populations. The basis for these similarities is apparent in the words and responses of survivors: The traumatic event has had a profound impact on their fundamental assumptions about the world.
>
> (Janoff-Bulman 1992: 51)

Janoff-Bulman argues that the immediate effect of a traumatic experience is the confrontation with one's own fragility. She writes:

> The confrontation with real or potential injury or death breaks the barrier of complacency and resistance in our assumptive worlds, and a profound psychological crisis is induced.
>
> (Janoff-Bulman 1992: 61)

This 'psychological crisis' is experienced as a sense of inner turmoil. The assumptions about the self and about the meaning of the world that had provided the background framework for the victim are shattered:

> Suddenly, the self- and worldviews they had taken for granted are unreliable. They can no longer assume that the world is a good place or that other people are kind and trustworthy. They can no longer assume that the world is meaningful or what happens makes sense. They can no longer assume that they have control over negative outcomes or will reap benefits because they are good people. The very nature of the world and self seems to have changed; neither can be trusted, neither guarantees security.
>
> (Janoff-Bulman 1992: 62)

For Janoff-Bulman the essence of trauma is in the way the inner world of the victim is abruptly ruptured and starts to disintegrate. They move from feeling safe in their world to feeling vulnerable. This brings about a 'double dose of anxiety' (her words). On the one hand the victim is overwhelmed with feelings of fear. Their world becomes intensely frightening. Their very survival may be in question. On the other hand their 'conceptual system' is broken and in a state of upheaval. Their fundamental assumptions, which provided security, coherence and order, are shattered. Janoff-Bulman gives the names 'terror' and 'disillusionment' to these two aspects of anxiety. She proposes that the symptoms of PTSD are best understood as being produced as part of the individual's innate attempts to cope with these feelings of terror and disillusionment. Cognitive processes that are not fully conscious, such as those described by Horowitz (see above), come into action and give rise to the intrusive-avoidance symptoms of PTSD. However, Janoff-Bulman also suggests that there are more conscious activities that victims characteristically pursue in order to rebuild their shattered assumptions:

> Cognitive strategies represent one extremely important means by which survivors facilitate this demanding reconstruction process. These are motivated cognitive strategies, not in the sense of conscious manipu-

lation, but rather in the sense that effect is strategic; they facilitate the
coping process by better enabling victims to reformulate a view of reality
that can account for the victimization and yet not be wholly threatening.

(Janoff-Bulman 1992: 117)

In addition, she calls attention to the importance of 'social support' in
aiding the recovery from trauma. As with the other approaches to trauma
discussed above, the social world is understood to be something external
to the individual victims. For Janoff-Bulman the social world is mainly
important because it enables individuals to receive 'feedback' about their
own behaviours and about the nature of the world. This feedback is then
internalized and enters a 'cognitive-emotional' equation, which becomes
the basis for a new assumptive framework.

Trauma, meaning and science

In the cognitivist framework traumatic events produce their effects by
clashing with the victim's internal schemas, the ways in which their
thoughts about themselves and the world around them are ordinarily
structured. After a traumatic experience the individual has to modify
his/her schemas to fit the new reality. They have to find new meanings for
themselves and their world. The intrusive-avoidance symptom complex is
understood to be the result of this process. These symptoms reflect the
desperate attempts of the individual to incorporate the new 'information'
involved in the trauma. Most researchers in the area of trauma are now
adherents of some form of cognitive approach.

The accepted understanding is that the centrality of the intrusion-
avoidance motif reflects this desperate search for meaning and order. For
Horowitz and others, this process is conceptualized as a purely internal
phenomenon located entirely within the confines of the individual self. It
is a process that can be understood scientifically and can be helped by a
series of technical interventions, which encourage the processing of the
traumatic material. While Horowitz acknowledges that there are social,
cultural and somatic aspects to the reaction to trauma, his approach is to
separate out the cognitive phenomena and focus upon these. Other
cognitive theories work in a similar way to this. These conceptualize the
social world in terms of 'social factors', discrete aspects of the
environment, which can be individually measured. Support from relatives,
friends and community is conceptualized in terms of 'social support
factors', which are then put forward as acting as 'buffers' or 'moderating
variables' against the impact of traumatic events. These social factors are
conceived of as acting on the individual 'from the outside'.

In the cognitivist framework the basic form of human psychology is held to be universal and not determined by social or historical context. Human reality is structured by psychological laws that can be scientifically investigated. While the *content* of cognitions and emotional states can be historically and culturally influenced, the way in which these cognitions and emotions are structured and ordered remains the same. Just as a database running on my computer will contain information relating to my work, and my neighbour can have the same program with completely different information, so too human beings, according to cognitivism, have the same programmes running with different content. Because of this, it makes perfect sense for researchers in this area to search for a 'unifying theory', an account of trauma that explains how all the different 'factors' relate and which can be empirically investigated. Lee and Turner make a typical call:

> A wholly persuasive model is required which offers an explanation of the complexity and range of the associated symptomatology. Also such a theory needs to answer why some people develop PTSD and others do not. Furthermore, no theory of PTSD can be complete without empirical data to back up the findings.
>
> (Lee and Turner 1997: 71)

Thus, in the current discourse of trauma we see a very good example of how cognitivist models work in the clinical area. This discourse incorporates all the markers of Cartesianism, identified in the last chapter: individualism, separation of mind from the 'outside' world and positivism. In addition, this discourse works with a traditional linear approach to the question of time and causality. In fact, the very diagnosis of PTSD makes a strong statement, in itself, about the nature of time. As Allan Young writes:

> PTSD is a disease of time. The disorder's distinctive pathology is that it permits the past (memory) to relive itself in the present, in the form of intrusive images and thoughts and in the patient's compulsion to replay old events. The space occupied by PTSD in the *DSM-III* classificatory system depends on this temporal-causal relation: etiological event → – symptoms. Without it, PTSD's symptoms are indistinguishable from syndromes that belong to various other classifications.
>
> (Young 1995: 7)

It is worth noting that much of the biological research in this area has been predicated upon this temporal-causal framework. Thus researchers have tended to assume the causal nature of the traumatic event and examine biological reactions to this. The traumatic event, or stressor, is understood to bring about pathological changes in an otherwise normally functioning physiological system. As we have seen above, *DSM III* PTSD represents a considerable shift in thinking about trauma compared to earlier accounts. Specifically, in *DSM III*, traumatic events come to be seen as causative factors in their own right. 'Normal' people, with no prior psychopathology, can be rendered severely ill by exposure to trauma. In the work of Horowitz, and others, PTSD is understood to be at the end of a continuum of 'normal' responses to frightening events. Biological researchers have used this paradigm and used animal models of responses to stress to investigate the biology of PTSD. As Yehuda and McFarlane note:

> The concept of an a priori biological response was an appropriate counterargument to critics who attacked the diagnosis of PTSD as having a political and philosophical origin, and it provided a post hoc scientific hypothesis that a biological response to trauma reflects a natural physiologic process.
>
> (Yehuda and McFarlane 1995: 1707)

In the next chapter I shall argue that this understanding of time and causality is proving inadequate to explain the biological research findings in relation to trauma. I shall suggest that a substantially different paradigm is needed.

Summary

In this chapter I have explored the concept of PTSD. After discussing the symptoms involved in the syndrome, as currently defined, I pointed out that PTSD is generally held to capture the central psychological sequelae after traumatic experiences. It is also assumed that it is valid cross-culturally and trans-historically. In the second part of the chapter I reviewed various conceptualizations of the disorder and argued that cognitive models are currently dominant. In the concluding section, I briefly pointed to the philosophical assumptions at work in these models. In the next chapter I will explore the limitations of the current discourse on trauma and suggest that some of the difficulties are philosophical in nature.

Chapter 4
The limitations of cognitive approaches to meaning and trauma

In the last chapter I discussed the current discourse on trauma within psychiatry and psychology. I made the case that cognitivism is very much at the heart of this approach and argued that this represents a crystallization of the modernist trend, which dominates these disciplines more generally. I used the term Cartesian to characterize the major underlying philosophical assumptions at work. I also noted a commitment to a linear approach to time and causality. This chapter looks at evidence that tends to contradict these assumptions. Although one of the themes of this book is a critique of PTSD and the discourse on trauma, it is important to acknowledge that the emergence of this discourse has had many positive results. In her book *Trauma and Recovery* (1992), Judith Herman argues that there is, and always has been, a tendency to push traumatic events not only out of individual consciousness but out of social consciousness as well. To study the effects of traumatic events, particularly such acts as rape, torture and sexual abuse, is to come face to face with the capacity for evil in human nature, and also to confront human vulnerability in the natural world. The tendency is to avoid such confrontation. She argues that:

> . . . to hold traumatic reality in consciousness requires a social context
> that affirms and protects the victim and joins victim and witness in a
> common alliance. For the individual victim, this social context is created
> by relationships with friends, lovers, and family. For the larger society,
> the social context is created by political movements that give voice to the
> disempowered.
>
> (Herman 1992: 9)

Herman argues that the discourse on trauma in the past 20 years has emerged because of a number of political developments, most importantly the rise of the women's movement in Europe and North America. The advent of feminism, she suggests, has made it possible for psychia-

trists to examine the effects of trauma and to take the victims' accounts of
their suffering seriously. She also suggests that the large-scale social
movements that opposed the war in Vietnam allowed for a critical examination of the effects of wartime experiences. Prior to this, government
propaganda and recruiting campaigns had been effective in promoting the
idea that the experience of battle and soldiering in general was somehow a
positive maturing influence on the individual. The fact that there was a
political campaign that looked upon the war in Vietnam as a negative
phenomenon meant that there was again a political context in which
psychiatry could take seriously the negative effects of wartime experiences. From Herman's point of view, PTSD has always existed but has
remained almost invisible to psychiatry until recently. Previous attempts to
explore it, such as the early work of Freud, were abandoned on account of
a lack of wider social support for such endeavours. Thus, for Herman, the
fact that trauma is now 'recognized' means that victims who were previously ignored will receive attention. It also means that the effects of rape
and domestic violence, of torture and warfare are taken seriously. Many of
the people who are currently involved in PTSD research and treatment
have a background in the feminist, anti-war and human rights struggles of
the past few decades. Often their involvement in the science of trauma
stems from an effort to provide legitimacy to political struggles. As we saw
in the last chapter this emerges very clearly from writing about how PTSD
came to be included in the *DSM* of the American Psychiatric Association in
1980.

However, in my opinion, the positive impact of the current discourse
on trauma in our society is undermined by the fact that it has been built on
certain assumptions – assumptions which carry a moral, cultural and
political weight, as we shall see later in this book. Before dealing with the
possibility that this discourse could be having a negative impact, both
within the Western world whence it sprang as well as in the countries of
the developing world to which it is now being exported, I wish to
highlight the problematic nature of the philosophical assumptions which
underlie it. These create a picture of meaning as something produced
within an individual's mind; this is held to be something internal, private
and solitary. The 'magic circle' of meaning is a personal creation. Trauma
wreaks havoc by interfering with the processes of this interior realm. It is
up to doctors, therapists and counsellors to rebuild the magic circle when
it is broken. I believe that these assumptions are challenged by a wide literature pertaining to the effects of violence and war. Positivism presents the
world of human thoughts, feelings and behaviours as something to be
researched and analysed along similar lines to the way in which the
sciences of physics, chemistry and biology have investigated the nature of

the physical world. Within psychology the positivist approach has served to marginalize the role of social and cultural context and their influence on an individual's mental state. Positivism renders the mind as having a given structure that can be researched independently of context. The assumption is that, as the mind is produced by the brain, and because this has basically the same structure in people everywhere, there is a universal form to human thought and emotion. Positivist psychology downplays the importance of history and culture and, in relation to trauma, asserts that PTSD captures the universal nature of human emotional reactions to violence and horror. The individualist focus of contemporary psychology has also led to a neglect of attempts to understand social and communal dynamics in the wake of trauma. Because it is assumed that meaning is generated within individual minds these dynamics have not been theorized as having a central role. As well as these positivist and individualist assumptions, contemporary psychology also works with a notion of linear causality. In what follows of this chapter I will present evidence that contradicts all three of these suppositions. I am arguing for a very different picture of how human beings exist with a sense of meaning in their lives. For me, the 'magic circle' is social through and through. It is something produced by our immersion in language, culture and social roles. We need an understanding of trauma that is adequate to this reality.

Individual reaction to trauma: historical aspects

While PTSD was first defined as an entity in 1980, since its formulation a number of researchers have claimed to find evidence that the syndrome has always existed. This is not surprising, given psychiatry's positivist self-understanding. Daly (1983) argues that the symptoms of PTSD are described in the famous diary of Samuel Pepys. In this, Pepys describes his experience of the Great Fire of London. His account of this begins on the 2nd of September, 1666. Pepys describes the gradual progression of the fire towards his home and details his own fear and the terror he sees in other people as they are unable to protect their property. He describes how he subsequently developed 'dreams of the fire and falling down of houses'. He was still unable to sleep 'without great terrors of fire' six months later. Daly suggests that Pepys' symptoms included intrusive images of his frightening experience, feelings of detachment, and memory impairment. The claim is that Pepys' diary establishes that PTSD (as defined by modern psychiatry) existed in the past.

O'Brien makes the point that several authors have championed this claim that 'PTSD is merely the renaming or the synthesis of an age-old condition' (O'Brien 1998: 5). He calls for caution, and in a review of various anecdotal papers that make this claim, found few which actually made a convincing case in its favour. While historically there is considerable evidence of physical and psychological reactions to terrifying events in the medical and non-medical literature, most of these reports point to symptom complexes that are *not* congruent with the defined symptoms of PTSD. For example, there are descriptions from the American Civil War of soldiers who developed symptoms of lethargy and withdrawal. These were thought to be due to 'nostalgia', in turn due to their being far away from home. There were also descriptions of syndromes such as 'soldier's heart' and 'irritable heart' which, whatever their aetiology, clearly manifested in physical symptoms located in the chest. The syndrome of 'shell shock' was described in the First World War. The symptoms of this were said to be the result of loss or impairment of the functions of the central nervous system and were assumed initially to be the result of organic damage (Mott 1919). The symptoms of shell shock have been variably described but included daze, fear, trembling, nightmares and an inability to function. Conversion hysteria was also commonly described in the First World War. The most common symptoms among British soldiers were: paralyses, contractures, muscle rigidity, gait disorders, seizures, tremors, spasms, blindness, muteness, fugue states and other symptoms of nervous system dysfunction. In addition to these syndromes, military doctors also described syndromes of 'neurasthenia' and 'disordered action of the heart'. In other words, the symptoms of shell shock are simply not the same as those of PTSD. In his book *A War of Nerves: Soldiers and Psychiatrists 1914–1994*, the military historian, Ben Shephard, writes:

> The experience of being shelled seemed to leave men blinded, deaf, dumb, semi-paralysed, in a state of stupor, and very often suffering from amnesia. Some could remember nothing between the moment of the explosion and coming in to hospital; others could remember nothing at all. A number of these patients also showed physical symptoms, such as extraordinary, unnatural ways of walking, that astonished the doctors who examined them in England.
>
> (Shephard 2000: 1)

The reader will see that this description is of a condition not grasped by the symptoms of PTSD outlined in the last chapter. Likewise, in the Second World War, there were a number of studies of symptoms associated with combat. Grinker and Spiegal (1945) documented the 19 most common symptoms that persisted long after soldiers were removed from combat. According to frequency of occurrence, the top five were restlessness, irritability, fatigue on arising, difficulty falling asleep and anxiety.

On reviewing these studies one is led to the conclusion that the symptoms of intrusion and avoidance, which are at the heart of the *DSM* concept of PTSD, actually figure quite infrequently. Somatic symptoms appear much more often. On this account, it is simply wrong to conclude that PTSD (as currently defined) has always existed. In spite of this, PTSD is often presented as though it was something 'discovered' by psychiatrists, something which, since being discovered, throws light on other unexplained areas of psychological functioning. In fact, the evidence would suggest that there has been a great deal of variation across history with regard to how people respond to horrible events. As we saw in the last chapter, Allan Young has argued that PTSD is something *created* by psychiatry at a particular historical and cultural moment. This is not to say that the suffering that the PTSD concept attempts to capture is in any way fictional or unreal. It is not to say that in the past people did not suffer in the wake of life-threatening, terrifying or deeply distressing events. It *is* to assert that the symptoms defined by the *DSM*, and the way in which they are grouped and related to one another, constitute one particular way of approaching and understanding the sequelae of such events.

The importance of social context: social and cultural dynamics in the wake of war and violence

The French sociologist Emile Durkheim noted that in the nineteenth century there was a widespread reduction in the suicide rate in those European countries affected by civil war. According to Durkheim (1951) the 'common enemy' acted as a source of social cohesion that in turn acted to lessen the isolation of individuals and diminish feelings of loneliness and depression. In the twentieth century, the suicide rate fell in nearly all European countries during the two world wars. At the outbreak of World War II it was widely assumed in Britain that one of the effects of the war would be an increase in the number of mental patients. Arrangements were made at the start of the war to receive large numbers of psychiatric casualties from the civilian population as the war began to involve urban communities (O'Brien 1994). Such people were subjected to terrifying bombing raids, food shortages, family bereavements and lack of sleep, all of which were thought of as causal, or at least participatory, factors in mental breakdown. However, following 15 months of continuous warfare there was found to be no increase in the admission rate in the Bristol area (Hempill 1941) and in Coventry there was a decrease in the attendance at the psychiatric outpatients. It was even argued that the war was having a beneficial effect on the mental health of many people, possibly because family and social life had become more intimate as entertainments, shopping, and travelling were restricted. Hempill expressed the view that 'the war has had little adverse effect on the mental health of the general population, and has been of benefit to certain types of individuals, especially women'. He noted a decrease in admissions to his mental hospital in the year 1941 and showed that, for those people who did attend for treatment, factors attributable to the war did not play a significant part in the reasons for admission. He wrote:

> The necessity of extending hospitality to neighbours, friends and the homeless seems to have brought reality closer to the shut-in mind: as one hypochondriacal woman said, 'You can't think of yourself when everyone is going through so much.'
>
> (Hempill 1941: 180)

During the Spanish Civil War large numbers of civilians were again involved. Furthermore, the enemies in this war were not from a different country with a different language, rendering them easier to 'dehumanize'. Rather they were fellow Spaniards, often from the same village or even the same family. Again it was assumed that in these circumstances there would be a significant increase in mental breakdown, but this proved not to be the case. In 1939, at the end of the war, Emilio Mira, Chief Psychiatric Inspector to the Spanish Republican Army, noted that the amount of psychiatric illness that developed during the war did not call for the provision of more psychiatric beds than had been available during peacetime. In addition he noted that:

> Depressed and neurotic patients whom I had looked after in private found relief in working for some public service – for example, social work. There was no increase in the average rate of suicide. I had the impression that many depressed and other mentally ill people were better when confronted with the actual demands and situations that arose during the war than when they were concerned only with their conflicts.
>
> (Mira 1939: 1219)

Closer to the present time, a number of studies have been reported from Northern Ireland, where a guerrilla war was waged for most of the past 30 years. In 1969 when the first riots broke out, an increase in psychiatric admissions or clinic attendance was expected. Not only did this not happen, but Lyons (1972) observed an actual decrease in the recorded rates of depression. He postulated that this was directly related to the outbreak of street violence, which allowed a discharge of aggressive impulses that otherwise would be inwardly directed, causing depression.[1] In a review of studies from Northern Ireland, Curran (1988) states:

> Judging from hospital referrals and admission data, suicide and attempted-suicide rates, the practices of psychoactive-drug prescriptions, and community-based studies . . . the campaign of terrorist violence does not seem to have resulted in any obvious increase in psychiatric morbidity.
>
> (Curran 1988: 470)

He suggests a number of reasons why the war has failed to produce a rise in observed psychiatric morbidity. In keeping with the work of Durkheim, Curran puts emphasis on the notion of increased social cohesion in times of war. He says:

> During rioting and other spells of sectarian disorder, followings killings of the most horrific nature, certain subpopulations and communities may bind together in a sense of common purpose and common outrage . . . Maybe, in the Belfast ghettos, there is a feeling of a real or indeed a supposed common enemy, whether it be the British, the Irish, the Catholics, the Protestants, the Army, the police or whoever. Identification and feeling 'one of us' against 'them' may defend each population and its members against overt psychological disturbance in the face of chronic civil disorder and tension, sectarianism, and acts of terrorist violence.
>
> (Curran 1988: 475)

Thus there is good evidence that wartime suffering and trauma is not inevitably associated with increased psychiatric morbidity. A common theme in the reports quoted above is the importance of social processes such as increased cohesion and solidarity in times of war. However, it would be wrong to assume that all wars are the same, or that all people in a given population are affected in the same way. The social position of women in many societies may mean that rape in wartime is something about which there is little discussion. There may well be substantial social stigmatization associated with rape and thus social cohesion will not extend to victims of sexual violence. In different ways, depending on social norms and expectations, this failure of solidarity and cohesion may affect others groups as well.

In a number of conflict situations, particularly in South America, there is evidence that oppressive states actually worked systematically to undermine social cohesion and solidarity, particularly during conflicts of the 1970s and 1980s (Jenkins 1991). For example, torture has been deliberately used (in preference to assassination) by such regimes, as simply killing a community leader may create a martyr for the community, a symbol of strength and resistance, while torturing such a person to the point where they are broken and scarred and then releasing them in a disabled state means that the person returns to the community injured, inarticulate and frightened. He/she has become a living symbol of the community's vulnerability and weakness (Ritterman 1987).

We can conclude that the social context in wartime profoundly affects the ways in which communities and individuals experience and react to the various traumas that violence brings. Social context can be supportive or destructive, have positive or negative effects. What I am emphasizing here is simply the fact that not only is social context *important* but it can also be the *most important* issue determining outcome.

Based on her work with Salvadorean women refugees living in North America, Jenkins raises questions about the validity of using the individual trauma model in cross-cultural situations. She argues that there is a need to look at 'collective trauma':

> Because traumatic experience can also be conceptualized collectively, person-centred accounts alone are insufficient to an understanding of traumatic reactions. In addition to the social and psychocultural dynamics surrounding any traumatic response, the collective nature of trauma may be related to what was . . . referred to as the political ethos characterizing an entire society.
>
> (Jenkins 1996: 177)

Jenkins suggests that accounts that start at an individual level will never be 'fully adequate in understanding traumatised cultures' (1996: 177). Derek Summerfield, a psychiatrist who worked for many years at the Medical Foundation for the Care of Victims of Torture in London, has published widely on this theme. He argues that the individualistic concept of PTSD cannot grasp the cultural dimension of suffering in times of war, particularly in non-Western settings:

> Western diagnostic classifications are problematic when applied to diverse non-Western survivor populations. The view of trauma as an individual-centred event bound to soma or psyche is in line with the tradition in this century for both Western biomedicine and psychoanalysis to regard the singular human being as the basic unit of study.
>
> (Summerfield 1997: 150)

Summerfield draws on a wide range of examples to make his point. For example, the war in Southern Sudan has not only caused lost of life and injury to individual victims, it has also destabilized a way of life:

> Disruption of the traditional cycle of animal husbandry resulting from
> the Sudanese civil war has brought social breakdown to the pastoralist
> Southerners. Cattle are crucial to them, being a form of currency not just
> in trading, but also in rituals and disputes. Tribal marriages can no
> longer be arranged because of dislocation and lack of cattle (the only
> traditional dowry) and women are driven to prostitution in the town,
> something previously unheard of. Because of the endemic killings and
> rape in the countryside, security conditions have become prime deter-
> minants of social behaviour, to the extent that families with noisy
> children are pushed out. Half this population has been forced to
> abandon villages regarded as ancestral places, seeking precarious safety
> in urban areas where their traditional skills are worthless. One study of
> teenagers displaced to Juba showed the resultant estrangement and loss
> of social identity: none could write a history of their clan and many did
> not even know the names of their grandparents or the village their clan
> came from.
>
> (Summerfield 1996: 6)

Summerfield, who has extensive experience of working with refugees in
London and has worked as a consultant with Oxfam in Rwanda and
Bosnia, argues that cultural factors are not only important in determining
the degree of disruption and dislocation facing individuals in times of war,
but culture also determines how people cope with their suffering and seek
help:

> . . . psychological trauma is not like physical trauma: people do not
> passively register the impact of external forces (unlike, say, a leg hit by a
> bullet) but engage with them in an active and problem-solving way.
> Suffering arises from, and is resolved in, a social context.
>
> (Summerfield 1996: 25)

The anthropologist (and psychiatrist) Maurice Eisenbruch introduced the
concept of *cultural bereavement* in 1991 in a deliberate attempt to move
beyond the individualistic discourse based on PTSD. Eisenbruch argues
that for many refugees and others displaced from their homelands and
home cultures loss of a known way of life is the *key* issue that determines
psychological and social outcome. In an empirical study he examined
differences between two groups of unaccompanied and detached
Cambodian adolescents. The first group were fostered in Cambodian
group care in Australia while the second group were living with foster
families, both American and Cambodian, in the USA. Eisenbruch found
that the cultural bereavement among those in the USA was significantly
greater than that found among those in Australia. In the latter context
there was less pressure to abandon the old way of life and the children

were actively encouraged to participate in traditional ceremonies. Many of the children who were fostered by American families in the USA saw little of other Cambodians and experienced little exposure to Cambodian culture. These children were in a precarious position psychologically, according to Eisenbruch, and displayed sustained feelings of regret at having lost their homeland. They continued to be immersed in the past and were preoccupied with thoughts of their families. Eisenbruch comments:

> The fieldwork showed that much good could be done by promoting access of the refugee children to Buddhist monks and Cambodian *kruu kmae* (traditional healers). It was striking how often my young Cambodian informants expressed their yearning to participate in traditional Buddhist ceremonies. They wanted to learn how to chant with the monks and the older participants, and how to 'make merit' for their dead or lost parents and ancestors for a better life in the next incarnation and to protect themselves from vengeful spirits.
>
> (Eisenbruch 1991: 674)

The importance of social context: culture and emotion

Cross-cultural studies of emotion have recently tended to undermine the positivist notion (discussed in Chapter 2) that emotional states have the same form universally and that these forms are independent of culture. I believe that it is becoming clear that culture mediates, in a very pervasive way, the experience and expression of emotion. Jenkins (1996) quotes Rosaldo's formulation of emotion as:

> . . . self-concerning, partly physical responses that are at the same time aspects of moral or ideological attitudes; emotions are both feelings and cognitive constructions, linking person, action and sociological milieu. Stated otherwise, new views of culture cast emotions as themselves aspects of cultural systems, of strategic importance to analysts concerned with the ordering of action and the ways that people shape and are shaped by their world.
>
> (Jenkins 1996: 168)

This has implications for the cross-cultural understanding of emotional reactions, including reactions to frightening or violent events. If culture shapes emotional experience in a pervasive and profound way, where does that leave the 'emotional processing' theories of cognitive psychology, and with them the current discourse on trauma?

The work of Jenkins, Summerfield, Eisenbruch and others takes us out of, and beyond, the individualistic focus of PTSD and the therapeutic concern with 'processing'. It is beginning to emerge with increasing clarity that if the individual trauma model works at all, it works in a culture with a strong individualist agenda. Most non-Western cultures do not work with such an agenda and so major practical difficulties arise when this model is exported. In spite of this a number of clinicians and researchers have continued to assert the universal relevance of the PTSD framework. Laurence Kirmayer points out that this model is attractive because:

> . . . it performs three great simplifications: (a) morally, it simplifies the issue of responsibility, guilt, and blame that plagues survivors and authorizes their righteous anger or forgiveness; (b) scientifically, it suggests a linear causal model amenable to animal models and simple experiments; (c) therapeutically, it allows clinicians to attribute a wide range of problems to a single wound and so to organize treatment along clear lines that may include both the moral and scientific models.
>
> (Kirmayer 1996: 155)

Kirmayer argues that there has been a neglect of somatoform and dissociative disorders in Western psychiatry in recent years.[2] He suggests that trauma can be 'inscribed on the body' in different ways and in many non-Western societies somatization and dissociation are the mechanisms most commonly involved. Kirmayer argues that:

> The mechanisms of the cultural shaping of symptomatology . . . differ in some details for somatic, anxiety and dissociative symptoms. Models of somatization emphasize somatic amplification and symptom attribution . . . models of anxiety emphasize cognitive evaluation leading to catastrophizing loops . . . models of dissociation involve alterations of attention, absorption in imagery, and attributions of involuntariness . . . (T)he specific social mechanisms posited . . . all involve a hierarchy of attentional mechanisms, attribution and interpretation, narratization, discourse, and praxis in which simpler psychophysiological processes are embedded in more complex levels of social meaning.
>
> (Kirmayer 1996: 149–50)

In other words, traumatic experiences will effect different responses in individuals, depending on the culture in which they live. Cultures differ in how they promote conscious and non-conscious ways of dealing with distress. Individuals experience and endure suffering in different ways and with different symptomatic outcomes:

> Thus the effort in the PTSD literature to isolate a simple cause-and-effect relation between trauma events and specific symptoms ignores the social and cultural embedding of distress that ensures that trauma, loss, and restitution are inextricably intertwined.
>
> (Kirmayer 1996: 150)

If Kirmayer's analysis is correct, then it would be safe to assume that the intrusion-avoidance symptom complex described in *DSM* PTSD, would have varying levels of significance in different societies. An empirical study carried out by the author of this book in Uganda provides some support for this conclusion (Bracken 1994). In the study, the author and a social worker from the same area interviewed 148 people from two neighbouring villages. These villages were in the Luwero Triangle, a part of Uganda that had suffered greatly during the war years. As part of the interview a number of questionnaires were used. One of these was the Impact of Events Scale (Horowitz et al. 1979) which seeks to measure the respondent's level of intrusive and avoidance symptoms. In addition, the social worker made an assessment of each individual's 'level of social functioning', using the Axis V scale from the *DSM III*. This is a measure of the 'highest level of adaptive functioning' over the preceding year. The score is determined after consideration of the person's functioning in terms of (a) social relations, (b) occupational functioning and (c) use of leisure time. It was found that intrusive and avoidance symptoms *were* reported when specific questions were asked about them. Furthermore, their presence was associated with the level of suffering endured during the war years. However, there was no association between these symptoms and the level of social functioning. In other words, those who had suffered most and who had the highest scores on PTSD symptoms were not necessarily the ones who had the poorest social functioning.

Similar results were reported from a study carried out in Nicaragua by Summerfield and Toser (1991). This research was of war-displaced peasants who were all survivors of atrocities. Summerfield commented on their results:

> I studied peasants displaced by war in Nicaragua, all survivors of atrocities, and found that features associated with post-traumatic stress disorder were common, but these people were nevertheless active and effective in maintaining their social world as best they could in the face of the continuing threat of further attacks . . . When these people did seek treatment it was for psychosomatic ailments, which are not included in the definition of the disorder . . . The diagnosis of post-traumatic stress disorder says little about ability to function.

> (Summerfield 1991: 1271)

Similar findings have been reported in Cambodian war refugees in the United States (Mollica et al. 1987). Thus, while the intrusive-avoidance symptom complex might be found in different settings this does not mean that it has the same *significance* in these settings. Depending on the cultural position of the people involved, other symptom complexes may be present and may be of more importance. In addition, the level of social functioning may be influenced by factors other than these PTSD symptoms. There are many aspects of human life that on initial inspection appear to be universal but which with greater attention and study are revealed to have different meanings within different cultures. For example, most people on the planet have a belief in some sort of deity. Superficially, it would appear reasonable to assert that religious worship and prayer show up as universals in human experience. Closer study reveals the weakness of this assertion. It tends to show great differences in the ways disparate people understand the relationship between their god(s) and human beings and the role of prayer and sacrifice in this relationship.

Likewise, nightmares do not have the same significance in all cultures and yet on a superficial level frightening dreams are reported universally. In a culture where dreams are not rigidly separated from waking reality and thus are endowed with great significance, threatening dreams may have a dramatic effect on waking beliefs and behaviours. In a culture where dreams are considered to be irrational and insignificant experiences it is rare for waking beliefs and behaviours to be modified in the light of such nightmares. This example is relevant to cross-cultural studies on trauma as nightmares are one of the most frequently reported 'intrusive' symptoms.

Trauma and linear causality

So far in this chapter I have presented evidence that the individual-trauma approach is severely limited in relation to cross-cultural work. I shall now look at two further difficulties for current models. The first problem concerns evidence that has emerged about the epidemiology of PTSD, the second concerns aspects of the biology of the syndrome. What is at stake here is the question of causation. The diagnosis of PTSD does not simply describe a number of symptoms but, importantly, also determines what has caused them. Even if other factors are understood to operate in bringing about these symptoms, the very logic of having a syndrome such as PTSD at all means that the person making the diagnosis is making a strong case in favour of some traumatic experience(s) having a causal link to the symptoms. We noted this issue at the beginning of Chapter 3. PTSD is one of the very few psychiatric diagnoses where the aetiology is identified in the diagnosis itself. As such it brings to the fore the under-lying assumptions about causality which operate in contemporary psychiatry and psychology. These have their origins in a particular strain of Enlightenment thought which developed the idea that the world (and ourselves) functioned as some sort of mechanism. We briefly discussed the model of linear time and causality in the last chapter. In his book *Time and Psychological Explanation* (1993) Brent Slife argues that this model underscores a great deal of theoretical and therapeutic work in psychology at present. While he does not deal with trauma specifically his arguments are relevant here.

Slife suggests that positivist psychology has used a notion of time and causality borrowed from Newtonian physics. He says:

> Attempting to establish itself as a science, psychology modelled not only the scientific method of Newton's physics but also the philosophy of Newton's *meta*physics. Central to both was Newton's rendition of linear time – absolute time. Although later physical scientists were to challenge, if not reject, this assumption, psychology essentially retains it.

> (Slife 1993: 7)

This is also a common-sense view of time and temporality in Western societies. Time is generally understood to be independent of mind and consciousness. It is 'out there'. Each moment is separate. The past is like a great collection of different moments. While we rarely question the nature of the metaphor involved, we accept that time 'flows' in some way and it does so in a linear fashion. The past comes before the present that is before the future. We usually think of memory as involving some sort of storage of the past. We saw in Chapter 2 how cognitive psychology uses a computer analogy to orient its theoretical endeavours. In Chapter 3 we examined the way in which this analogy has been used in work on trauma. In a great deal of this work trauma is understood to overwhelm the mind and create a block in the mind's ability to process information. Memories from the past continue to intrude upon the present. Slife makes the point that a number of cognitive researchers have acknowledged that memory involves more than a simple storage of memories. They accept that when remembering we do not passively retrieve data from storage but actively reconstruct associations and memories from memory fragments. However, he argues that as they continue to theorize from within an empiricist framework they continue to work with a linear notion of time and causality. Schemes that are said to do the work of reconstruction are themselves products of previous experiences encoded in the mind in different ways. Thus, 'even explanations that seem to emphasize present or reconstructive aspects of cognition are often reducible to conventional linear theorizing' (Slife 1993: 117).

As with the positivist approach to the question of meaning, discussed in Chapter 1, time and memory are presented as 'things' existing in the world. Time is a determinate entity and memory can be measured and analysed. Events happen in time that is basically a series of moments. Memories, however produced, are re-presentations of past events. The basic theory of PTSD is premised upon this way of thinking about time. The separation of past and present is *built into* the diagnosis. If we use the diagnosis of PTSD we are implicitly making a strong case for this separation; it simply doesn't work without it!

Questions from empirical PTSD research

Traditional accounts of PTSD present a rather simple scenario: an individual, who carries the weight of a particular history, experiences a traumatic event. This is extremely stressful and the individual develops characteristic symptoms that are indicative of certain processes taking place within. Social factors impinge on these processes and can facilitate or interfere with their progress but do not determine their essence. The response to traumatic events is understood to be an exaggeration of the physiological and psychological response to stress. Thus animal models of stress reactions should be useful in understanding the human biology of PTSD.

In different ways the problems that have emerged concern the 'flow of time' in this account. In the original PTSD framework the characteristic symptoms are understood to be a reaction to the trauma. This motif clearly underscores Horowitz's account and the thinking behind the *DSM III* version. The traumatic event happens first, then the symptoms emerge. We noted in the last chapter that the big innovation involved in the concept of PTSD was its proposal that the trauma *was the aetiology* of the syndrome. This proposal distinguished *DSM III* PTSD from earlier accounts of post-traumatic reactions. It also distinguished PTSD from other psychiatric syndromes with similar symptoms such as depressive disorders and obsessive-compulsive states. It was assumed that empirical studies would confirm the validity of this formulation.

In the original formulation of PTSD the role of the stressor was seen as obvious and clear-cut. *DSM III* merely states that to make the diagnosis there should be: 'The existence of a recognizable stressor that would evoke significant symptoms of distress in almost anyone'. The epidemiological evidence about PTSD after disasters and other 'obviously traumatic' events calls this assumption into question. In fact it would appear that the development of PTSD after a significant trauma such as combat or rape is the exception, rather than the rule. Estimates of the prevalence of PTSD after a criterion A stressor event are given in *DSM IV*.[3] They are said to range from 3 to 58 per cent (APA 1994). One of the major studies of Vietnam veterans found a 15 per cent prevalence of current PTSD and a 30 per cent lifetime prevalence (Kulka et al. 1990). Of those exposed to the

Mount St Helens volcano eruption, only 3.6 per cent developed PTSD symptoms (Shore et al. 1989). After reviewing such studies, Yehuda and McFarlane comment:

> . . . in documented epidemiological studies it is difficult to find even transitory symptoms in more than 50% of the population, and in the majority the symptoms will have usually resolved within 2–3 years. Thus, the available epidemiological data show that PTSD, and certainly chronic PTSD, is more unusual than usual following exposure to a variety of traumatic events.
>
> (Yehuda and McFarlane 1995: 1708)

The McFarlane quoted above is an Australian psychiatrist who, in the 1980s, studied a large group of firefighters who were exposed to very traumatic events in the course of a major bush fire. These traumatic events easily met the original PTSD stressor criterion. McFarlane had access to the men's psychiatric records and he followed them up with interviews and questionnaires over an extended period of time. He has reported on a number of conclusions. Severity of exposure was not the most important factor determining symptomatic outcome. Only a small number of the men, described as 'anxiety-prone', developed characteristic intrusive and avoidance symptoms. Indeed, 'pre-morbid vulnerability accounted for a greater percentage of the variance of disorder than the impact of the disaster' (McFarlane 1989: 227).

Allan Young discusses McFarlane's findings at some length in his book *The Harmony of Illusions.* Young argues that not all of those who develop symptoms after a traumatic event do so in a way that corresponds to the *DSM III* formulation. Thus, a certain number of people will develop significant psychopathology, but in them post-traumatic symptoms are not *triggered* by the trauma. Instead, anxiety and depressive symptoms are induced by the traumatic event. These then bring into being the PTSD intrusion-avoidance symptoms: 'Once anxiety symptoms and/or depression have become established, a *feedback effect* begins to occur where the intensity and frequency of the memories of the disaster are increased' (McFarlane, quoted in Young 1995: 138).

McFarlane's research was based on people who developed 'rapid-onset PTSD', in other words they became symptomatic very quickly after the trauma. The likelihood is that their anxiety or depression *was* induced by the events. However, Young makes the point that if we accept that anxiety or depressive states can bring about the intrusive-avoidance symptoms of PTSD *at all*, then we have to accept the possibility that at least some cases of delayed-onset PTSD are induced by anxiety or depressive states which occur *independently* of the actual event, which then becomes the focus of these intrusive-avoidance phenomena. In other words, Young interprets McFarlane's research as opening up the possibility that in some cases of PTSD the 'flow of time' does not correspond to that incorporated in the *DSM* concept of the disorder. This has very serious implications for research on PTSD. The two sorts of case, i.e. one where the symptoms emerge from the event, the other where preoccupation with the event is the result of the prior emergence of other symptoms, cannot be distinguished by phenomenology alone, nor even by presence/absence of a stressor. This ambiguity, about time and causality, is hopelessly engrained into the very definition of PTSD. As we saw in Chapter 3, more recent versions of the *DSM* have indicated an awareness of the complexity associated with the stressor criterion and it has been described differently in post-*DSM III* versions. However, PTSD remains *defined* as a syndrome in which symptoms flow *from* the event. Those situations where the flow is in the other direction simply cannot be accommodated, and so are ignored. Part of this problem, at least, stems from the model of time and causality operating within traditional accounts of PTSD. As I shall show in our discussion of Heidegger's philosophy, in the next chapter, he presents an approach to temporality in which simple distinctions between past, present and future cannot be made. For an approach developed from Heideggerian phenomenology the causal ambiguity identified in traditional PTSD research serves, not as a problem, but as a *support* for the theory.

PTSD is also presented, in current models, as involving an exaggeration of the normal stress response. This was clearly the guiding assumption of the work of Mardi Horowitz. The assumption was quickly made that animal models of stress reaction could be used, unproblematically, to investigate the human biology of PTSD. Initial results appeared to confirm this.[4] However, more recent findings suggest that the symptoms of PTSD are associated with biological phenomena that are *not* a reflection of the normal biology of stress. For example, researchers looking at hypothalamic-pituitary-adrenal (HPA) axis alterations in PTSD have found results that are at odds with those found in the 'normal' stress literature. Yehuda et al. (1995) summarize research in this area as follows:

> The findings suggest that, rather than showing a pattern of increased adrenocortical activity and resultant dysregulation of this system, individuals who suffer from PTSD show evidence of a highly sensitized HPA axis characterized by decreased basal cortisol levels, increased number of lymphocyte glucocorticoid receptors, a greater suppression of cortisol to dexamethasone, and a more sensitized pituitary gland compared to individuals without PTSD. Thus, in addition to the classic pattern of increased cortisol levels in response to stress, there may be a

contrasting paradigm of cortisol abnormalities following stress, characterized by diminished cortisol levels as a result of stronger negative
feedback inhibition. This paradigm compels us to expand the stress
response spectrum.

                                                    (Yehuda et al. 1995: 362)

Like the epidemiological research findings quoted above, these findings
point to the conclusion that human responses to trauma are simply more
complex than initially proposed in the *DSM* formulation of PTSD. In
particular, they tend to support Young's suggestion that the direction of
causality in post-trauma psychiatric syndromes is ambiguous. Yehuda et al.
remark: 'To the extent that PTSD is conceptualized as a stress disorder, the
findings challenge us to regard the stress response as diverse and varied,
rather than as conforming to a simple, unidirectional pattern' (1995:
362–63).

Summary

In this chapter I have argued that the current discourse on trauma is
simply inadequate to grasp the complexity of how different human beings
living in different cultures respond to terrifying events. There are
problems with attempts to understand trauma as an event impacting on an
individual in isolation, problems with models of emotions that separate
these from cultural context, and problems with the assumption of linear
causality that underscores the very concept of PTSD. My argument is that
all these difficulties emerge from the Cartesian philosophical framework
that underscores modern psychology and psychiatry.

I believe that cognitive models of mind and positivist psychology
more generally are severally limited in their ability to describe the actual
worlds inhabited by human beings. These models work with assumptions
of individualism, positivism and linear time. Cognitivists attempt to fit our
experiences into these models much like Victorian women attempted to fit
their bodies into corsets. From the evidence discussed above it would
appear that the model of PTSD is currently working like a psychological
corset. It has had some success in drawing our attention to the suffering of
victims of different kinds but because of its underlying assumptions it is
unable to grasp the complexity of this suffering.

The dominant model of PTSD, predicated upon a cognitivist
framework, suggests that the intrusive-avoidance symptom complex is
associated with a loss of meaningfulness in the life of the victim after the
traumatic experience. For example, in the work of Janoff-Bulman,
examined in the last chapter, traumatic experiences are said to 'shatter the
assumptions' held by the victim about themselves and the nature of the

world. If Allan Young is correct and, in some cases at least, the flow is the other way around, then the implication is that vulnerability with regard to meaningfulness may not simply be the *result* of trauma but might, in some way, be a predisposing factor for the development of problems after such events.

The analysis presented here points to the fact that, in reality, the situation is far more complex than originally proposed in the *DSM* account of PTSD, as the contexts in which people endure traumatic experiences differ greatly. However, almost the entire biological and psychological research literature on PTSD, as an entity, has been carried out from within the traditional framework and works with its assumptions. We should not expect this literature to provide *direct* support for a framework that works with a very different approach to human reality, such as that presented in the next section. However, the points of contention *within* the traditional PTSD literature, I believe, point to a degree of complexity in the area of trauma which the traditional approach cannot easily accommodate, and thus support the need for an alternative approach to human reality, meaning and trauma.

A phenomenological approach
to meaning and its loss

Chapter 5
Heidegger's account of human reality

Introduction

In this section, I move to the central concern of the book: the relevance of Heidegger's philosophy to contemporary problems in psychiatry and, in particular, to the question of meaning. My aim is to open up a different theoretical approach to the world of mental illness and to show how Heidegger can be of help in this endeavour. As a result these chapters are more theoretical than the last two and I hope the reader is not put off by this. Having used the discourse on trauma to show how the current assumptions of psychiatry work in practice and having pointed to major difficulties with this I shall now attempt to demonstrate the pertinence of Heidegger's thought to this issue. I want to show how the sort of hermeneutic phenomenology developed by Heidegger offers us a very different framework for understanding the way we experience our world as being meaningful and how this sense of meaning can be lost.

In this chapter, I outline the Heideggerian alternative to Cartesianism. By now the reader should be familiar with the assumptions of Cartesianism and understand how these work to shape the theory and practice of psychiatry. The aim of this chapter is to engage directly with these assumptions. The chapter is in two parts. The first part focuses on the contrast between Heidegger's notion of 'being-in-the-world' and the Cartesian separation of mind from world. In the second part, I go on to outline Heidegger's critique of scientific reductionism and positivism and discuss his approach to temporality. I use this critique to challenge the cognitivist understanding of meaning and, in particular, the concept of 'intentional causality' developed by Bolton and Hill (see Chapters 1 and 2).

In the traditional psychiatric framework, disorders are defined and theoretically modelled as a first step. Then therapeutic techniques are developed and tested. The notion of cultural particularity only emerges as a sort of 'afterthought' when these models and techniques are being applied to people from non-Western societies. In Heidegger's philosophy human beings are *always* temporal, embodied[1] and culturally situated[2], *always* linguistically and historically located. In a psychiatry organized around the concept of 'being-in-the-world' (see below), contextual issues are foregrounded. They become the first step.[3]

Following on from this, Chapter 6 is centred on Heidegger's collaboration with the Swiss psychiatrist, Medard Boss. This includes a discussion of the seminars given by Heidegger for a group of psychiatrists at Boss's home in the years between 1959 and 1969. I also discuss Boss's own attempt to bring Heidegger's insights directly to bear on the clinical world of medicine and psychiatry. I want to show how Boss used insights from Heidegger in a positive way but I also want to show how his approach was limited because he failed to really get away from the framework of psychoanalysis. In Chapter 7, I discuss Heidegger's writing on the issue of anxiety and its relationship to meaning. I argue that this opens up a different perspective on the problem of trauma. Finally, in Chapter 8, the last part of this section, my concern is to get beyond what I see as some of the limitations of Heidegger's early thought. This opens the way for a discussion of postmodernism and postmodernity in Section III.

Heidegger: a controversial thinker

Heidegger was born in 1889 in the small German town of Messkirch, in the state of Baden. He spent most of his life in this region and owned a small cabin in Todtnauberg, in the nearby Black Forest. This was his place of retreat and he would retire there at regular intervals throughout his life. He studied philosophy with Husserl at the University of Freiburg and later, after some years in Marburg, he himself held the chair of Philosophy at Freiburg. He died in 1976.

Heidegger remains a controversial thinker, mainly because of his association with Nazism in the 1930s. This was a significant involvement and cannot be ignored as a minor aberration. Heidegger became a major advocate of National Socialism and the 'führer principle' in the world of higher education. In his biography, Rüdiger Safranski says that Heidegger was 'bewitched by Hitler' (1998: 232).

How much Heidegger's philosophical thought is implicated in his disastrous political involvement is open to debate. On the one hand, the insights of *Being and Time* clearly cannot be dismissed as some sort of crude Nazi metatheory. On the other hand, there is undoubtedly an affinity between Heidegger's talk of 'authenticity' and 'resoluteness' and the Hitlerite calls for commitment to the cause of national salvation. In his thoughtful introduction to Heidegger, George Steiner writes:

> The evidence is, I think, incontrovertible: there *were* instrumental connections between the language and vision of *Sein und Zeit*, especially the later sections, and that of Nazism. Those who would deny this are blind or mendacious. In both – as in so much of German thought after Nietzsche and Spengler – there is the presumption of, at once mesmerized by and acquiescent in, a nearing apocalypse, of so deep a crisis in human affairs that the norms of personal and institutional morality must be, shall inevitably be, brushed aside.
>
> (Steiner 1978: 117)

Safranski (1998) provides a comprehensive account of Heidegger's politics. For a very short but helpful discussion of the issue I would recommend Jeff Collins's *Heidegger and the Nazis* (2000). My own view is that Heidegger's philosophy opens up new ways of thinking about ourselves as individuals and social beings. He disturbs our (culturally embedded) common-sense assumptions. He raises interesting and challenging *questions*. This is all to the good. However, given what we know of his politics we should be wary of his *answers*. If we follow Heidegger's thought at all we should be clear where we break away from him. I am particularly uncomfortable with his contrast between 'authentic' and 'inauthentic' modes of life. This is where I part company. I shall return to this in Chapter 8.

I Heidegger's critique of individualism and 'internal' accounts of mind

Being-in-the-world

Traditionally, both philosophy and psychology begin theorizing with a mind relating to a world outside it. This is their starting point. The major challenge for both has been to understand how these two realms (mind and world) are connected. However, it is clear that for the most part we live our lives without assuming that we have a mind that relates to an outside world at all. We simply get on with things. Having the thought that there is a mind relating to a world outside is a *theoretical* move. It is a thought that only becomes possible when we stand back from our practical involvement in life. This practical involvement is primary, more basic. To be human is to be involved, implanted, immersed in the everyday world. Heidegger wants to engage with human experience at this more basic level, at a level before we have moved to a theory involving separation.

In fact, he wants to philosophize in the opposite direction: away from notions of 'mind', 'world' and 'representation'. This can be difficult for us in the modern era, not least because the very language we use to describe our experience has Cartesian assumptions built into it. In an attempt to get beyond this language Heidegger uses composite terms such as 'being-in-the-world'. He wants to avoid the usual way of thinking about how we are *in* the world. We are not in the world in the same way that my cornflakes are *in* their box or in the way that a brain resides *inside* a skull. It is ourselves who give meaning to the world that we inhabit: we *construct* our world as we live in it. In some ways we are responsible for allowing a world to be in the first place. And this world must be different for us as humans from that of other animal species. The way in which human bodies are made anatomically and physiologically means that a certain type of world 'opens up' for us. Humans have a certain way of hearing, seeing and smelling the world, a certain way of experiencing space and time. We bring colour and sound to the world. It is difficult for us to imagine what sort of world 'opens up' to a fruit fly, a fish or to a bat. We are simply not 'in' a world that is separate from ourselves. Rather, we allow a world to be by our very presence. Heidegger uses the composite term 'being-in-the-world' in an attempt to describe the complexity of our involvement with our worlds. He says:

> Being-in is not a 'property' which Dasein has and sometimes does not have, and *without* which it could *be* just as well as it could with it. It is not the case that man 'is' and then has, by way of an extra, a relationship-of-Being towards the 'world' – a world with which he provides himself occasionally.
>
> (Heidegger 1962: 84)

> . . . this structure is something 'a priori'; it is not pieced together, but is primordially and constantly a whole.
>
> (Heidegger 1962: 65)

Traditional ways of thinking about ourselves as minds 'containing' representations of an outside world fail to grasp the 'a priori' nature of this structure. There simply is no world incorporating sights and sounds, outside, waiting to be represented. Heidegger seeks a very different vocabulary to describe our reality.

The concept of Dasein

The way in which a world 'opens up' for us is not just dependent upon our physiology. A human world only becomes possible to us because we live in that world with other people and in the midst of a culture. The opening up of a world is never an individual act. When I look at a flower and see it as red and beautiful I can do so only because my human physiology allows me to see (or reveal) a certain part of the electromagnetic spectrum and make contrasts with other colours. But it is also possible only because I have the idea of a flower and the notion of beauty available to me. I experience the world with words, beliefs, emotions and patterns of thought that come from the social world in which I live. Human reality is both individual and social at the same time. Again, Heidegger introduces a new word to describe this complexity. He says that we exist as Dasein, 'being there'.[4] Dasein is different from all other ways of being because humans exist and relate to their world in a way that no other entity does. Human existence is qualitatively different from that of rocks and stones, plants and animals. Dasein, *human* being, involves an openness to all things, including itself. Indeed, as McCall puts it, 'human being is open being' (McCall 1983: 70). Charles Scott, in a discussion of the work of Medard Boss (see next chapter), says that: 'human being is irreducible, perceptive world-openness' (Scott 1975: 183). As far as we know, humans are the only creatures on our planet that are 'open' in this way. Not only does a world show up for us but we aware of our role in this. We are aware of the world as a totality. We can think about time and its origins. We can imagine our own death and thus the passing of a world. In short, in Heideggerian terms, we are open to the question of being. We are ontological.

Heidegger also characterizes Dasein as a *Lichtung*. The word *Lichtung* usually refers to a clearing in the woods (according to Macquarrie and Robinson, the translators of *Being and Time*). The noun *Licht* also means light. These translations convey a sense of things in the world being revealed, an opening being made, through the illumination provided by Dasein: humans bring about a 'disclosing' of the world. As pointed out above, the world that is disclosed through us is (presumably) very different to that which is available to other creatures. While this is an act of individual humans, it is never this alone. As Dreyfus puts it:

> We can thus distinguish *clearing* as an activity from *the clearing* that results from that activity. Think of a group of people all working together to clear a field in a forest. There is a plurality of activities of clearing, but all this activity results in only one cleared field.
>
> (Dreyfus 1991: 165)

When we open our eyes and ears we see a world around us. As Heidegger maintains, this act of perception is never passive: it is also an act of creation. We 'bring into being' the colours, shapes and sounds of the world. Furthermore, we experience the world, not as a collection of discrete items, but as a totality, something that 'holds together'. We experience it as meaningful. But we do this as a social group, not as a collection of individuals. Thus, any individual act of perception has a social dimension. It is dependent on our human physiology but also on our social embeddedness: our involvement in a world socially ordered through human practice, language and culture.

Heidegger's reversal of the Cartesian cogito

Heidegger's term, Dasein, therefore incorporates the notion of a fundamental lack of separation between ourselves and the world in which we live. Heidegger criticized Descartes, not only for separating mind from world but also because for Descartes, human subjectivity became a *res*, a thing, just another entity in the world. We saw this in Chapter 2. Louis Sass says:

> Such a way of thinking obscures the essential inseparability of consciousness and its objects . . . Heidegger considers this tendency to interpret, understand, or express ontological issues concerning the fundamental nature of the world on the analogy of empirical facts within the world . . . to be the deepest and most treacherous source of confusion in the entire history of Western thought.
>
> (Sass 1992b: 292–93)[5]

For Heidegger, human subjectivity is not just another entity in the world but is instead the transcendental ground of the world. It allows a world to be.

Not only is Dasein always being-in-the-world, according to Heidegger, but we are in fact 'thrown' (*geworfen*) into the world. We do not know whence we came into being, he says, nor do we know towards what end (apart from inevitable death) we have been projected into existence. We simply find ourselves in the midst of the world, involved in it. The world is always already in us as we are always in it. Our orientations within the world are thus prior to any consciousness we may have of them. Reflection, of any sort, always takes place in the context of a worldly embedded life. It is never, and can never be, primary. Traditional Western philosophers, even before the Cartesian cogito, have put the notion of reflection first, arguing that it is through reflection that we get to the world, to reality. However, for Heidegger we are always *living* our lives before we start to reflect. Our practical involvement comes first. Philosophically, if we are to comprehend anything about our place in the world we have to return to our everyday involvement with things. Objects in the world are primarily seen as tools, equipment, instruments. In order to understand a hammer, for example, we need to know how to hammer, how to use it. When we do this, Heidegger maintains, the detached reflective stance is seen for what it really is: a secondary, derived position. The separation between consciousness and the object (such as the hammer) that appears so self-evident to a philosopher who is sitting back in an attitude of reflection or observation, is not at all in evidence when one is actually using the object. It is at those times when we do not feel wrapped up in our surroundings, when the hammer breaks or when we feel bored or we daydream, that we begin to reflect and ultimately to philosophize.

Thus Heidegger stresses our pre-cognitive, pre-reflective involvement with the world. Dasein is 'always already' involved and the world is always primarily 'ready-to hand' (*zuhanden*), and as such it is always already meaningful prior to any reflection. Descartes and Kant began their reflections with the assumption of disconnection between mind and world (in Descartes this had an ontological dimension). They then sought to find instances of epistemological connection which were certain and secure. By starting with the notion of Dasein as already in the world Heidegger actually reverses the direction of the problematic. Thus, in the Heideggerian framework what needs to be explained is not the connection, which is the basic given, but the instances of disconnection. Such instances of disconnection occur when we are interrupted in our practical, cognitive or emotional involvement with the world and we find ourselves in the position of reflection.

This position allows Heidegger effectively to reverse the Cartesian cogito, which confidently asserts the primacy of detached thought: '*cogito ergo sum*' (I think, therefore I am). For Heidegger the reverse is the case: 'I am, therefore I think.' Existence, in the sense of lived human existence, involved and embedded in the world, is the necessary precedent and the enabling condition of thought. George Steiner writes:

> Platonic-Cartesian cogitation and the Cartesian foundation of the world's reality in human reflection are attempts to 'leap through or across the world' (ein Uberspringen) in order to arrive at the noncontingent purity of eternal Ideas or of mathematical functions and certitudes. But this attempted leap from and to abstraction is radically false to the facticity of the world as we encounter it, as we live it.
>
> (Steiner 1978: 86)

Meaning and intelligibility

Heidegger's reversal of the cogito has important ramifications. For our purposes it has implications for the philosophical assumptions of cognitivism and the question of meaning. Perhaps most importantly it challenges the underlying assumptions of the Cartesian and 'rationalist' tradition that locate our ability to experience the world as meaningful in the cogito: our thought about the things of the world. For Heidegger, the background intelligibility in which entities show up at all, and do so as particular types of entities, is given *firstly* by our practical engagement with the world. As we have seen above, this is dependent both on the fact of our embodiment and our involvement in a social world. Dasein's clearing activity is something that cannot be grasped simply in terms of mental representations, concepts or schemas. We 'dwell' in the world in a practical way. We *know how* to get around in this world before we *know about* it. We are orientated in our worlds in ways that cannot be made completely explicit. We have an understanding of our world that cannot be completely formulated. Knowledge (cognition) is a specialized mode of being-in-the-world. This is the difference between his version of how the world is meaningful and that of the Cartesian and other rationalist philosophies.

Charles Taylor puts forward the notion of 'engaged agency' in an effort to tease out the implications of Heidegger's perspective. He says:

> . . . the dominant conception of the thinking agent that Heidegger had to overcome was shaped by a kind of ontologizing of rational procedure. That is, what were seen as the proper procedures of rational thought were read into the very constitution of the mind and made part of its very structure.
>
> The result was a picture of the thinking agent as disengaged, as occupying a sort of protovariant of the 'view from nowhere', to use Nagel's suggestive phrase. Heidegger had to struggle against this picture to recover an understanding of the agent as engaged, as embedded in a culture, a form of life, a 'world' of involvements, ultimately to understand the agent as embodied.
>
> (Taylor 1993: 317–18)

It is worth examining how Taylor works with the concept of embodiment to tease out some of the implications of a reversed cogito as developed by Heidegger.[6] Taylor begins his argument by making the point that the idea that the world of the agent is shaped by his or her body is actually generally accepted. However, there are two distinct ways in which we can understand this shaping. On the one hand, my experience is shaped in psychophysical causative fashion. Thus, as a perceiving agent I cannot see the wall behind me. This can be explained in causal terms. The light coming from the wall cannot reach my retina because the back of my head is in the way and my retina is pointed in the wrong direction. The physical, material characteristics of my body make my seeing the wall impossible. In this way my perception is shaped by my embodiment. My world is shaped by it.

A completely different notion is involved when shaping is understood as the provision of context and background so that my experience as agent becomes intelligible. This is a Heideggerian way of understanding the concept of one's world being shaped. For example, as I take in the room around me, even *before I think* about it, the scene already has a structure for me. It is already orientated for me. Some things are 'up', some things 'down'. Some are 'near', some are 'far'. Some objects 'lie to hand' while others are 'out of reach'. My world is shaped by my embodiment in the sense that this is the world of an agent with this particular kind of body. It is an agent who can move and deal with things in certain ways:

> To understand what it is to 'lie to hand' one has to understand what it is to be an agent with the particular bodily capacities that humans have. Some creatures from another planet might be unable to grasp this as a projectile term. Of course the creature might work out some descriptions that were roughly extensionally equivalent. But to project this term the way we do, one has to understand what it is to be human.
>
> (Taylor 1993: 319)

Thus there are two distinct ways in which we can understand the shaping of our experience by our embodiment. The first can be stated in causal terms. The second type of relationship is more in the way of a relating of the background facts of our embodiment:

> These two senses in which experience is shaped by embodiment help to explain the dialogue of the deaf between critics and exponents of artificial-intelligence-inspired theories of the mind. The former . . . have often insisted that the computer offers a model of 'disembodied' consciousness. Proponents of the artificial intelligence model, insulted in the very heart of their materialist commitment, generally find this accusation unintelligible. But it is easy to see why the criticism is not understood. Proponents of strong artificial intelligence are thinking of the first kind of relation. The second kind has not swum into their conceptual ken, and hence they have great trouble understanding what they are being accused of.
>
> (Taylor 1993: 334)

Thus embodiment provides the pre-cognitive, pre-reflective lived experience that is the condition of intelligibility for any statements about ourselves. The nature of our embodiment, as context or background, can be described but cannot be made fully explicit. Embodiment is known implicitly. We have what Heidegger calls a 'pre-understanding' (see Taylor 1993: 327) of what it is to act as humans. Dreyfus says:

> Such an understanding is contained in our knowing-how-to-cope in various domains rather than in a set of beliefs that such and such is the

case. Thus we embody an understanding of being that no one has in
mind. We have an ontology without knowing it.

(Dreyfus 1991: 18)

Thus the background meaning and intelligibility of our world is something
we experience in the context of our bodily and practical engagement with
that world. It is not 'generated' by detached thought. Indeed it provides
the context in which thought about entities can happen at all.

The point is that the world is meaningful for us in a way that defies
formulation. It has a background coherence and intelligibility that cannot
be grasped through an analysis of constituent elements. It is 'given' to us
as embodied social creatures. Proponents of artificial intelligence and
cognitive psychologists deny this and seek to make explicit the processes
through which we make sense of the world. Heidegger understands the
intelligibility of the world as 'holistic'.

A couple of examples may help. Any act of perception involves
something appearing against a background in a figure–ground
relationship. Gestalt psychologists have analysed this relationship at
length. We perceive the figure through its distinctive features. These can
be described and are determinate. The ground, on the other hand, is
essentially indeterminate. It cannot be grasped in descriptive terms.
Dreyfus says that the ground can only be understood as 'that-which-is-not-
the-figure' (Dreyfus 1994: 240). Brent Slife quotes this comment from
Dreyfus in his critique of the linear time assumptions of cognitive
psychology. He argues that the holistic nature of human perception and
meaning-making undermines the validity of information processing
models which all involve some sequential characterization of these
phenomena. He says:

> This means that the ground *cannot* be formalized. The surrounding
> context of the figure cannot be positively described, let alone specified
> in the precision necessary for a linear processing machine. If it is
> attended to or examined, then *it* becomes the figure and the ground is
> lost again.
>   . . . The upshot is that artificial intelligence cannot, in principle,
> operate like human intelligence. Information processing requires a
> reductionism of the information that loses the holistic qualities of the
> parts, and many of those holistic qualities, such as the ground of percep-
> tions, cannot be formalized for linear input.
>
> (Slife 1993: 134–35)

Another example is the way in which we find music meaningful. To the
majority of humans, music is experienced as something important,
something purposive, something meaningful. We are able to appreciate

music because our biological nature is of a particular kind. We have the means to hear and to make sense of sounds. We can appreciate variations in tone and tempo. But music is also cultural. What sounds melodic to me might sound like noise to someone from a different culture. Growing up in any particular society, we are tutored from an early age to find particular rhythms and sounds of significance. Thus music is experienced as meaningful because of our embodied, encultured being-in-the-world. What is important here is the fact that this sense of meaningfulness cannot be explained by any analysis of the musical experience in terms of sub-elements. In his introduction to Heidegger, George Steiner uses the example of music to bring out the way in which meaning cannot be 'explained away' by science. He says:

> Is melody the being of music, or pitch, or timbre, or the dynamic relations between tone and interval? Can we say that the being of music consists of the vibrations transmitted from the quivering string or reed to the tympanum of the ear? Is its existence to be found in the notes on the page, even if these were never sounded . . . Modern acoustical science and electronic synthesizers are capable of breaking down analyt-ically and then reproducing any tone or tone-combination with total precision. Does such analysis and reproduction equate with, let alone exhaust, the being of music?
>   The answer eludes us. Ordinarily, we search for metaphorical description. Wherever possible we consign the question to technicality or to the limbo of obviousness. Yet we *know* what music *is*. We know it in the mind's echoing maze and in the marrow of our bones. We are aware of its history. We assign to it an immensity of *meaning*. This is absolutely key. Music *means* even where, most especially where, there is no other way whatever to paraphrase this meaning, to restate it in any alternative way, to set it down lexically or formally.
>
> (Steiner 1978: 47)

As we shall see later in this book these different approaches to under-standing how the world is meaningful for us have important implications for how we respond to situations where this meaning is at stake. If meaning is something produced in our worlds through schemas, thoughts or mental representation then it makes sense to engage with these mental phenomena in efforts to re-establish an ordered and coherent world. It makes sense to probe the contents of the mind in an effort to fix the faulty 'information processing'. This is the orientation of most forms of psychotherapy. On the other hand, if Heidegger, Dreyfus, Taylor and Slife are right, then the restoration of meaning requires, as a first step, a focus on the practical world through which a sense of order becomes available to us. Meaning in this frame is something generated holistically through our embodied engagement with a social world. If meaning is broken it will be through this social engagement that it will be restored.

In summary, human being, according to Heidegger, is always engaged being, embodied being. Human reality is always in the world and the world is always involved in that reality. It is impossible to conceive of any human existence that is not engaged thus. Our sense that we have an interior mind that exists in relation to an outside world only arises when we attempt to cease our involvement and start to reflect in a detached way. Such detachment is, according to Heidegger, actually impossible and we only have the sense of separation because our culture and the prevailing philosophical attitude assert that it is a fundamental aspect of human nature.

II Heidegger's critique of scientific reductionism and positivism

Significance

We have noted above Heidegger's argument that reflective thought is derivative and secondary to the practical involvement of Dasein in the world. One of his most original and important insights relates to the derivative nature of traditional concepts of the natural world, nature, in a number of different ways:

> Nature is itself an entity which shows up within the world and which can be discovered in various ways and at various stages.
>
> (Heidegger 1962: 92)

Primarily we encounter nature in 'available' forms: iron tools, wood, etc. as part of our practical involvement with the world. In this way, natural objects form part of our human environment and are useful, beautiful, harmful, and so on. But for the scientist, water (for example) shows up as atoms of hydrogen and oxygen. It has certain physical properties. It is not beautiful or refreshing. The scientific understanding of the natural world is achieved only by ridding it of such qualities. 'Worldliness' is Heidegger's term for the underlying environmental context in which Dasein exists. The scientific mode of our relating to nature only arises when we deprive '"the world of its worldliness" in a definite way' (Heidegger 1962: 94). Only by stripping the world of its values for us do we engage with it scientifically. We remove its significance and re-contextualize it in scientific theory. These processes 'produce' a nature that is understood in causal terms. Such is the work of the natural sciences.

Because philosophy has traditionally regarded detached reflective thought as our primary mode of involvement with the world the derivative nature of the natural science project has not been noticed by scientists or philosophers. This detached mode of thought 'passes over' the 'world' of being-in-the-world. In the traditional ontology dating from Descartes:

> The Interpretation of the world begins, in the first instance, with some entity within-the-world, so that the phenomenon of the world in general no longer comes into view.
>
> (Heidegger 1962: 122)

To get to the scientific view of reality we have to strip the world of its significance for us as individuals and as members of a community. This is what it means to be objective. But the world as significant is actually primary and the scientific position is derived. We seem to forget this. As a result, the scientific position has come to be seen as somehow more real, more basic. Because of this it has seemed plausible to propose the possibility of explaining the world, including the human world, in the terms of natural science. Thus emerged the positivist agenda. Heidegger's demonstration of the primacy of worldliness however brings such a project into question. He says:

> Even if (traditional) ontology should itself succeed in explicating the Being of Nature in the very purest manner, in conformity with the basic assertions about this entity, which the mathematical natural sciences provide, it will never reach the phenomenon that is the 'world'.
>
> (Heidegger 1962: 92)

His point is that because we produce the natural science concept of nature by stripping the world of human significance it is unlikely (to say the least) that we could reverse the project and explain significance in terms of such a dehumanized nature. Harrison Hall writes:

> Heidegger argues that this practical world, the intentionality appropriate to it, and the sense things have for us within it are more fundamental than the traditional sense of the world as a collection of things in objective space, the intentionality of cognitive acts, and the sense things have for us within such acts. That priority or fundamentality comes to at least the following:
>
> 1 The practical world is the one we inhabit first, before philosophising or engaging in scientific investigation – in Heidegger's words, it is where we find ourselves 'proximally for the most part'.
> 2 The world in the traditional sense can be understood as derivative from the practical world, but not the other way around – that is,

starting from Heidegger's account of the practical world we can
make sense of how the traditional sense of the world arises, whereas
any attempt to take objective perception and cognition as basic and
construct the practical world out of the resources traditionally
available is doomed to failure.

(Hall 1993: 128)

Human values are built into the world and are implicit in the skills with
which we involve ourselves with people and things. They are part of our
embodiment and involvement in a culture. In terms of embodiment,
experiences such as pain, pleasure, hunger and sexuality provide a
'valued' orientation towards the world but this orientation cannot be
stated explicitly because such values are not always open to cognitive
formulation. Such embodied experiences arise in particular human
settings and have significance only in such settings. Their significance
exists because of the background embodied and 'encultured' context in
which they occur. For Heidegger such significance is primary and cannot
be reduced to explanation in terms of a secondary derived theory. He
argues that explication of the realms of human significance, of 'worldliness', is only properly undertaken in a hermeneutic mode. The causal
explanatory framework of the natural sciences is singularly unsuited to the
task.

Some interpreters of Heidegger, most notably Dreyfus and Taylor,
have argued that his analysis reaffirms the Diltheyan distinction between
the natural and the human sciences: a clear distinction between the two
types of investigation in terms of what counts as appropriate methodology.
For them the investigation of the natural world within a causal explanatory
framework is valid but the human realm needs to be understood in
hermeneutic terms alone. Both Dreyfus and Taylor have used Heidegger's
work to support this approach. Their basic assertion that human beings
are unique, in being self-interpreting, is most clearly developed by
Heidegger in *Being and Time*. They contrast this with the position of
objects in the natural world that are not seen as having this self-interpreting quality. Both Dreyfus and Taylor are mindful of the post-empiricist
challenge to the status of natural science. In this, philosophers of science
such as Kuhn, Hesse and Feyerabend have argued that natural science is *in
fact* not the sort of neutral, objective, detached discipline that it was once
understood to be. Instead they argue that all natural sciences are loaded
with assumptions and exist in social and historical contexts that determine
their priorities and agendas to a large extent. As such, they all involve a
hermeneutic dimension. The implications of this development in the
understanding of scientific theory and practice are not underestimated by

Dreyfus and Taylor. Taylor, in a now famous quotation, summed up the irony involved:

> Old-guard Diltheyans, their shoulders hunched from years-long resistance against the encroaching pressure of positivist natural science, suddenly pitch forward on their faces as all opposition ceases to the reign of universal hermeneutics.
>
> (Taylor 1980: 26)

However, both philosophers have worked hard to maintain the distinction. They have presented various arguments to underscore the difference between the two. For example, Taylor has argued that although the natural sciences are also interpretive, the human sciences have to be doubly interpretive. This is because not only are the human sciences involved in interpretation but the objects of their study are themselves involved in self-interpretation. This does not hold in the natural sciences.

All of the arguments presented by Dreyfus and Taylor involve the Heideggerian notion of human being as interpretive. They contrast this with the ontologically distinct position of the natural world. They suggest that Heidegger's presentation of the derivation of the concept of nature in the scientific framework supports their view. However, an alternative interpretation of Heidegger is used by Joseph Rouse (1987) to support his critique of these neo-Diltheyan arguments. Rouse argues that the hermeneutic circle as elaborated by Heidegger radically undermines the Diltheyan position:

> Traditional Diltheyan hermeneutics emphasized the meaningful character of the *object* of interpretation, and the hermeneutic circle involved an interplay between the object as a meaningful whole and the parts that both compose the whole and acquire their sense from it. For Heidegger, the hermeneutic circle is an interplay between the *understanding* of the world as the meaningful configuration within which things are manifest as what they are and the *interpretation* of particular things within the world. The circle thus has the same structure for the interpretation of persons and of things, because it has nothing to do with the presumptively meaningful character of the object.
>
> (Rouse 1987: 182)

Thus, nature only 'shows up' in relation to Dasein. Rouse does not argue for an anti-realist position but aligns himself with the pragmatist position that the 'world *is* what shows up in our practices' (1987: 165). From this perspective what count as things, relations, or causes do so only within particular social and cultural contexts.[7] Not only is the social world constructed through human practice and language but so too is the very concept of nature. Thus, Rouse argues that Heidegger offers a way of being grounded in particular human circumstances:

> To say with Heidegger that only Dasein is meaningful is not to say that only human beings 'have' meaning, but rather to say that a practical, purposive configuration of world is the condition for anything's having any intelligible properties of any sort. Meaning is a 'formal' condition of the intelligibility of beings rather than a substantive characteristic of some particular being.
>
> (Rouse 1987: 183)

In spite of Rouse's usage of Heidegger's understanding of hermeneutics he is also critical of Heidegger's 'early philosophy of science'. He argues that this account presents science as essentially a theoretical activity that disengages the scientist and the objects of science from local, functional situations. In contrast, Rouse presents science as a practical, experiment-orientated activity that never manages to disengage itself from its social and political context. He says that Heidegger failed to give adequate attention to the actual practices involved in scientific research. Science is always, according to Rouse, 'local knowledge'.

These arguments concerning the proper relations between the natural and human sciences do not affect the argument developed above that human significance cannot be understood in terms of a dehumanized nature. Rouse, Taylor and Dreyfus all agree with the basic Heideggerian argument that human reality can only be understood in a holistic way. Significance is always generated against a broad background of linguistic structures and social practices. As such it can only be grasped and understood in relation to such background structures and practices. These are always multiple and unformalizable. Thus, understanding of human significance always requires a hermeneutic element. The attempt to generate human significance solely within the framework of a dehumanised natural science is thus doomed to failure. As pointed out in Chapter 4 Dreyfus has demonstrated this in relation to artificial intelligence (AI) models of mind. He says the practical failure of AI research to develop convincing models of human activities is practical support for Heidegger's position:

> It is easy to say that to account for the equipmental nexus one needs simply add more and more function predicates and rules describing what is to be done in typical situations, but actual difficulties in AI – its inability to make progress with what is called the common-sense knowledge problem, on the one hand, and its inability to define the current situation, sometimes called the frame problem, on the other –

suggest that Heidegger is right. It looks like one cannot build up the phenomena of world out of meaningless elements.

(Dreyfus 1991: 119)

In his recent book *The Undiscovered Mind: How the Brain Defies Explanation* (1999) the science journalist John Horgan provides a useful survey of the current state of psychiatry, psychotherapy and neuroscience. Horgan, unlike most other journalists writing on these subjects, stands back from the current mood of celebration and takes a cold look at what has actually been achieved. His conclusions are damning. He argues that after years of neuroscientific research we are nowhere near an understanding of how our minds work. He says that there is an 'explanatory gap' between neurophysiology and psychology which appears to be unbridgeable. He also speaks of the 'Humpty Dumpty' dilemma:

> It plagues not only neuroscience but also evolutionary psychology, cognitive science, artificial intelligence – and indeed all fields that divide the mind into a collection of relatively discrete 'modules,' 'intelligences,' 'instincts,' or 'computational devices.' Like a precocious eight-year-old tinkering with a radio, mind-scientists excel at taking the brain apart, but they have no idea how to put it back together again.

(Horgan 1999: 23)

Intentional causality

The arguments developed above hold even in relation to the sort of 'sophisticated' cognitivism put forward by Bolton and Hill (see Chapter 1). They argue the case for a psychological science which, while sharing a great deal in common with biology, cannot be reduced to the forms of explanation that exist in physics and chemistry. Psychology and biology are said to exhibit 'intentional causality', and explanations in these sciences require 'intentional explanations'. These are explanations that incorporate notions such as 'normal/abnormal', 'information', 'design', 'mistake' and 'rules'. According to Bolton and Hill, this terminology cannot be 'reduced' to the terminology of physics and chemistry. DNA and the haemoglobin molecule are put forward as exhibiting intentional causality, as well as such things as human thought and reason. The transitions between the two levels are said to be 'seamless' (1996: 260). Because of this it is appropriate to talk in terms of a 'predictive' science of psychology, albeit one which pays attention to human meanings. While they reject the idea that human reality can be explained by reference to 'physical laws', they nevertheless assert that cognitive psychology is in the business of establishing 'natural laws' and 'norms of function' in the mind.

They write, unproblematically, about people who develop psychotic episodes as possibly exhibiting a 'design fault' (1996: 284). If psychology can describe what the 'normal design' of a human being actually consists of, and can describe 'norms of function', then it can predict what will happen under particular conditions, given that the system is functioning 'normally'. They are quite clear that once such norms are established, psychology becomes a true causal science. They maintain:

> . . . the idea that the causal status of cognitive explanations derives from their place within a well-entrenched systematic empirical theory about relations between stimuli, cognitive states, and behaviour. There is something correct about this suggestion, but it is not yet complete. It omits special features of descriptions of functional systems, namely, that they essentially invoke *norms* of function, and that this accounts for their necessity.
>
> (Bolton and Hill 1996: 200)

Asserting that there are 'norms of function', which can be established, leads Bolton and Hill to elaborate an account of human beings as 'rational agents'. Unless human beings act in a rational and consistent way, the predictive power of psychology starts to evaporate. Because of this, they are led to propose that there are 'laws of reason', according to which particular behaviours can be judged to be rational or otherwise. Thus:

> If a person believes such-and-such, then she *must*, in appropriate circumstances, act in a way that accords with that belief. This 'must', however, has nothing to do with scientific theory or natural law. If the consequent of the hypothetical fails, no scientific theory has been refuted, still less has there been a miracle! Rather, the inference would be that, for one reason or another, the person has apparently acted irrationally. The nomological character of the prediction pertains to the 'laws' of reason, not to laws of an empirical science.
>
> (Bolton and Hill 1996: 201)

The problem with this theory is that there simply are no universally accepted 'laws of reason'. There are only human judgements about what it is to be rational or irrational. Anthropologists have long debated the supposed universal nature of rationality. Hobart (1985) describes how Balinese epistemology is highly sophisticated and subtle. He argues that in Balinese culture, language is recognized as polysemic, 'double-edged', and always influenced by the interests and intentions of both speakers and listeners. Truth is always relative to context. Hobart writes:

> Balinese ideas of what is manifestly so or not so cannot be grafted onto our model of propositions being true or false. Scepticism over human

abilities sets the Balinese sharply apart from Hellenic, and later, traditions of the omnipotence of reason.

(Hobart 1985: 113)

If this is the case, and complex and different rationalities exist in different
cultures, it is very difficult to see the value of talking about 'laws of reason'
at all. Any proposed set of 'norms', 'rules' or 'laws' of thought will always
be the product of a particular perspective. This is the central difficulty with
the approach of Bolton and Hill. While they claim to endorse a 'post-
empiricist' epistemology, they appear to locate this epistemology solely in
the *subjects* of psychological research, and not in the *researchers*
themselves. What a researcher puts forward as 'normal functioning' may
well be uncontentious and generally agreed in the world of biology, but
disagreement about the nature of normality is the *usual state of affairs* in
the world of psychology and psychiatry.

Bolton and Hill admit that generalizations in the area of human
psychology are 'vague' and 'non-specific' (1996: 207). Nevertheless, they
argue that such generalizations do exist and can be used scientifically. For
example, they quote the work of Seligman on the phenomenon of
'learned helplessness'. Seligman's original work was with animals, but the
concept of learned helplessness has been widely used as a model for
depression in human beings. Bolton and Hill argue that 'the cognitive-
affective state of helplessness [which] results from persistent or traumatic
(perceived) lack of control over major aversive events, such as pain, or
deprivation, and ensues in behavioural inertia' (1996: 206) is an example
of a generalization over a cognitive-affective state. This 'learned
helplessness' which results from negative life-events is understood by
many to lead to a state of intense hopelessness and, through this, is held to
account for many features of the syndrome of depression. Presumably this
would be an example of what Bolton and Hill mean by 'intentional
causality'.

In a similar vein one could develop 'causal' theories about the origins
of depression from the work of Brown and Harris. The Sri Lankan anthropologist, Gannanath Obeyesekere, quotes the following passage from
their work:

> The immediate response to loss of an important source of positive value
> is likely to be a sense of hopelessness, accompanied by a gamut of
> feelings, ranging from distress, depression, and shame to anger.
> Feelings of hopelessness will not always be restricted to the provoking
> incident – large or small. It may lead to thoughts about the hopelessness
> of one's life in general. It is such *generalization* of hopelessness that we
> believe forms the central core of depressive disorder.
>
> (Brown and Harris 1978: 134)

However, Obeyesekere makes the following observation:

> This statement sounds strange to me, a Buddhist, for if it was placed in
> the context of Sri Lanka, I would say that we are not dealing with a
> depressive but a good Buddhist. The Buddhist would take one further
> step in generalization: it is not simply the hopelessness of one's own lot;
> that hopelessness lies in the nature of the world, and salvation lies in
> understanding and overcoming that hopelessness.
>
> (Obeyesekere 1985: 134)

In other words, hopelessness is not something that has a fixed meaning.
How it relates to sorrow and loss is determined by cultural context. Thus
the relationship between life events, states of helplessness and
hopelessness and the syndrome of depression cannot be stated in terms of
an acultural, decontextualized law. States of depression can be interpreted
in terms of life events, but such interpretations emerge in the context of a
particular culture which places certain values on affective states and differ-
entiates such states in particular ways.

Similar observations have been made by Janis Jenkins and Marvin
Karno in relation to the concept of 'expressed emotion'. This is, currently,
one of the most researched constructs in psychosocial research and is
cited by Bolton and Hill. High 'expressed emotion' in the families of
patients with schizophrenia is understood to be causally related to relapse
in such patients after they leave hospital. However, Jenkins and Karno
demonstrate that there are substantial cultural influences on the way in
which family context, symptoms and relapse are related. Because most
researchers in this area of research are committed to psychology as a
causal science they have assumed the generalizability of the 'expressed
emotion' construct and failed to see the cross-cultural difficulties:

> Quite striking from a cross-cultural psychiatric point of view is the
> neglect on the part of expressed emotion researchers in calling for a
> systematic examination of the relationship between culture and
> expressed emotion. Since the anthropological and cross-cultural psychi-
> atric literature of the past several decades has documented substantial
> cultural differences in conceptions of psychosis, display of emotion,
> behavioral rules and norms, and family structure and identification, it is
> reasonable to expect that features such as these are of key relevance to
> the explication of expressed emotion. In our view, it is these features
> that go to the very heart of what the construct of expressed emotion
> embraces.
>
> (Jenkins and Karno 1992: 19)

One can only speak confidently about 'norms of function' and 'rational
action' in the human world, after one has bracketed out contextual

phenomena such as culture, language, gender, social and political circumstances, etc. However, according to hermeneutic philosophy (and most
anthropologists) these phenomena actually *constitute* the meaningful
reality of human beings. When one enters debates about cultural norms,
beliefs and practices, and how these relate to metaphysical and
ontological assumptions, one has *de facto* moved away from any sort of
causal framework. This is a realm of interpretation and hermeneutics.
Agreeing with Wittgenstein's characterization of psychological activity as
essentially 'rule-following', Harré and Gillett, in their book *The Discursive
Mind* (1994), argue that:

> Where this involves socially or culturally mediated content (as most
> human thought does), the rules embed shared norms. But rule-
> following is an inherently paradoxical activity. In being trained to follow
> a rule, a person is equipped with a disposition to respond to certain
> conditions in certain ways but is not causally compelled to do so.
>
> (Harré and Gillett 1994: 120)

Bolton and Hill convincingly argue that biological science involves a
strong element of 'functionality' that cannot be reduced to the terms of
physics and chemistry. However, the question being posed here is: to what
extent have they been effective in developing a conceptual bridge between
biological systems and lived human reality? As we have seen in the last
section, the Heideggerian argument is that the scientific account of the
world is produced by systematically stripping the language we use of
human value terms. It is a move away from the 'ready-to-hand' reality
within which we live, to another way of ordering the world. Positivism
seeks to use this 'de-valued' language of science to explain the nature of
lived human reality. As Bolton and Hill argue that biology can only 'work' if
we do *not* 'de-value' our language completely, and continue to use terms
such as 'normal', 'information' and 'mistake', it is not really surprising that
their version of biological reality has certain affinities with the human
reality from which they are borrowed. But this position is nothing less
than a tautology. Their failure to engage with the position of the observer,
the one who decides what is 'normal' or 'faulty' and writes the theories of
biology and psychology, renders their account unstable and open to the
sort of hermeneutic critique developed above in relation to more traditional forms of positivism.

Temporality and historicality

Before ending this chapter, I wish to examine Heidegger's approach to
time. Just as Dasein is always situated in a world of significance, so it is also

always temporal. In fact, according to Heidegger, it is because Dasein is temporal that a world of significance opens up at all. The title of Heidegger's great work emphasizes the importance of time. For him, a fundamental ontology is one in which being is shown to be inseparable from 'temporality' (*Zeitlichkeit*). In the introduction to *Being and Time*, he says:

> We shall point to temporality (*Zeitlichkeit*) as the meaning of the being of that entity which we call 'Dasein'.
>
> (Heidegger 1962: 38)

There is a close relationship between the way Heidegger approaches the question of Dasein's being-in-the-world and Dasein's temporality. In both cases there are established philosophical and common-sense under-standings of the relationship that Heidegger wants to oppose. Dasein is not in a contingent relationship to time, but rather temporality is part of its very make-up. Dasein 'temporalizes'. His account of temporality runs contra to the traditional philosophical approach to time dating back to Plato. In this tradition, time is modelled on a spatial metaphor, in which it becomes possible to be 'in time' or 'outside time'. To be outside time, to be atemporal, is to be in a transcendental relationship to the world and to Dasein.[8] By invoking a viewpoint on the world that is atemporal the human imagination exalts itself and reaches out of its embeddedness. Olafson says:

> The distinction between what is in time and what is not has been deeply entrenched in the Western philosophical tradition since Plato. That distinction treats what is not in time as superior, both intrinsically and for the purposes of knowledge, to what is in time. This Platonic conception of knowledge as directed ultimately to what is timeless became the model for the Christian idea of God's mind and knowledge. God himself was taken to be outside time, so his knowledge was in no way qualified by a temporal position. Instead, he knew everything, including things in time, in a timeless manner. In Heidegger's view, this conception of God's knowledge became, in the modern period, the model for understanding human knowledge.
>
> (Olafson 1987: 77)

In the traditional account, the notion of an atemporal vantage point is combined with a vision of time itself as a linear phenomenon. Time is understood to be a series of moments, a series of 'nows', each essentially disconnected from each other. While Aristotle conceived the 'now' as having a certain 'thickness', modern thought has sought to model the 'now' in atomistic terms. It is only from outside the series of nows that what is past, present and future can be established. Furthermore, the necessity of a possible atemporal position is also required to explain how any individual has a sense of his/her own position in time. In the model of linear time the person who is in time knows the past through representations. But there is a difficulty here as these representations are always present. Thus it is not clear how the person can reach out of the present and establish certain representations as being of the past and then relate to them as such. Why is it that all representations do not simply collapse into the present? This is only avoided by postulating an atemporal position from which it is evident which representations are in the present and which are from the past. In some way it is understood that the person who is in time has access to the atemporal viewpoint. This model is obviously problematic and has caused a number of difficulties for philosophy. However, the postulation of an atemporal position is often an implicit rather than explicit element of the model and so the problematic usually does not come to light. Modern common sense and psychology simply assume a clear distinction between what is present and what is past.

The notion of an atemporal vantage point is deeply entwined with the positivist notion of causality discussed in Chapter 2. Causal laws are understood to exist as 'hard and fast' unchanging connections between things. Such laws, by definition, do not change with time but work at different times and in different situations. As the psychologists Faulconer and Williams assert:

> The positivist notion of causality . . . relies on the assumption that static, atemporal entities are the fundamental kind of existing things and that other things exist only to the degree that they can be reduced to these static entities and their atemporal characteristics. Causal explanation is explanation in terms of these atemporal entities. In this sense causality *is* atemporality; the causal account is the atemporal one, and it is the only account by which human being is intelligible according to the positivist point of view.
>
> (Faulconer and Williams 1985: 1182)

Heidegger contradicts this by pointing out that time is at the essence of human being. To be human is to be temporal, involved in possibility and change. Without the presence of possibility no *human* event can really occur. Dasein relates to itself and to the world in a temporal way and cannot be grasped in terms of atemporal, static causality.

'Now', like the word 'there', is an indexical term. It works to date and locate events in the world by reference to the time at which it is *used* and thus to the person who uses it. In the traditional account, this indexicality is seen as an interference and attempts have been made to establish a non-indexical set of time concepts such as objective metric time. Heidegger rejects this move and with it rejects the linear notion of time. For him, just as the scientific concept of nature is *produced* by an active stripping away of value terms from the language in which we contemplate nature, so too our notion of linear time is *produced* by stripping temporality of its indexicality. In the traditional account human beings have a sense of the past, the present and future because they have access to a transcendental atemporal point from which events show up as being in time. Heidegger reverses this and argues that it is only because Dasein is temporal and as such has a 'built in' understanding of the movement of time that it then becomes possible for Dasein to imagine an atemporal position. In other words the notion of linear time and non-indexical time concepts are only possible because Dasein always already has a sense of change and a sense of past, present and future.

Heidegger argues that we have to stop thinking about the 'now' as a self-contained independent moment, existing as logically distinct from the past or the future. His move is to point to the internal complexity of the 'now' as it is actually experienced. For Dasein, the now is not simply a point in a series but rather it holds, or frames, time in such a way as to set up contrasts within itself between the past, present and future. Olafson says:

> Another way of putting this is to say that, in the Now, time is stretched (*erstreckt*) in such a way that it holds on to what has been and awaits something that is to come. The former is thus taken as that which is no longer, the latter as what is not yet; and what is now the case is present in the strong Heideggerian sense of that term as what once was not and later will (or may) no longer be the case. If what is now the case were simply replaced in the next moment by something else, then in each of these moments what is the case would be a Now without a contrasting Then, a present without a past or a future. But there is a future only if what is not yet the case is something other than just a state of the world that is located, for some transcendental and nontemporal observer, further along the time dimension.
>
> (Olafson 1987: 85)

As we have discussed above, Dasein is in a relationship of 'care' (*Sorge*) to the world and this relationship implies a continuity. In his discussion of care, Heidegger writes:

> The formal existential totality of Dasein's ontological structural whole must therefore be grasped in the following structure: the Being of Dasein means ahead-of-itself-Being-already-in-(the-world) as Being-alongside (entities encountered within-the-world).
>
> (Heidegger 1962: 237)

Thus Dasein discloses a world because of its particular make-up. In Heidegger's analysis there are three essential elements to how Dasein discloses. Human reality is structured as it is because Dasein is always:

1. *ahead-of-itself*: this is evidenced in our understanding. In this we are always thinking ahead in some way or another, always projecting into the future.
2. *already in*: this is evidenced by the fact that we are always already disposed to the world in some particular way. This is manifest through our moods or states of mind (*Befindlichkeit*, see next chapter).
3. *alongside*: we are always present to and involved in the world around us.

He says:

> The 'ahead-of-itself' is grounded in the future. In the 'Being-already-in
> . . .', the character of 'having been' is made known. 'Being-alongside . . .'
> becomes possible in making present.
>   (Heidegger 1962: 375)

The essential point being made is that the present is not and cannot be something that is separate from the past and the future. The three are involved inextricably with one another. This is seen clearly if we attempt to imagine a person existing in the present tense alone, without access to a past or future. It is simply impossible to imagine such a state. Our worlds are always already configured for us and this configuration implies a past. It makes no sense to think of a present moment in which the world is not configured in some way. Likewise, it makes no sense to think of a present without a future. It is akin to attempting to think of night without a concept of day, or vice versa. By speaking about a present at all we are implying the existence of something else, we are implying a movement onwards.

   Olafson discusses the implications of this approach for the notion of memory. He points out that memory is usually thought of in terms of 'episodic acts' through which we somehow reach out of the present into the past and through this we have access to representations of some previous events. In addition, the representations that are so recovered are often thought of, particularly in cognitive frameworks, as having been 'stored'. We thus carry them with us all the time but only retrieve them at certain moments. In this account the present is given a highly privileged position. It is from the present that we reach out and encounter our memories. This account of memory gives us a picture of a strong present which carries the past with it, stored away but accessible.

Olafson points out that this picture is problematic:

> What this misses, of course, is the way this supposedly present world
> bears a burden of pastness that is not at all a mere external supplement
> that a helpful memory is constantly adding to an otherwise rigorously
> present state of affairs. The identities in terms of which we understand
> and deal with the things and places and artefacts in our world are not
> construed on the basis of such a rigorous distinction between present
> reality and added information about the past . . . If we are to be thought
> of as carrying our pasts with us, the place where we 'store' them is the
> world, not our heads. We move and act and live within a world that is
> instinct with pastness; and although it is true that we do on occasion
> suddenly recollect things that we had forgotten, that recollection itself
> occurs within a world that is itself historical – that is, a world in which
> what happens (geschehen) happens in a present that has a past and a
> future.
>
> (Olafson 1987: 87)

Thus Dasein always and everywhere inhabits a world that is historical, a
world that is structured, ordered, and orientated in the past. For Dasein,
in an ironic way, the present *is* its own past. Just as the notion of 'stored
memory' cannot do justice to the way in which lived Dasein experiences
the past's involvement with the present, so also the notion of prediction
does not properly grasp the way in which the future is involved with
Dasein's present. Many, if not most, of Dasein's actions and thoughts
involve an element of futurity. In many ways Dasein's present is pregnant
with its future. The future is not something contingently related to the
present, rather every present is committed to a future. Dasein's existence
is primordially orientated towards the future and possibility:

> The primary meaning of existentiality is the future.
>
> (Heidegger 1962: 376)

For Heidegger the spatial metaphor in which we understand ourselves to
be 'in time' confuses the true nature of our temporality. For him Dasein is
not 'in time' as the entities of the world are, rather Dasein is the entity that
has time.

Summary

Heidegger offers us a way of understanding the human world which is
very different from that presented by Descartes and other philosophers
who have followed his strongly 'subjectivist' orientation. Richard Polt
(1999) makes the point that the world as described by Descartes is

'impoverished'. The Cartesian version of our reality is limited and fails to grasp the complex way in which our embodiment and practical engagement are involved in disclosing a world that is orientated and meaningful. Heidegger does not set out to disprove the Cartesian cogito but by adopting a phenomenological perspective reveals that our reality is simply richer than that allowed by the Cartesian approach. His critique of Descartes is made by showing the limitations of the cogito.

His philosophy can help us to ground a critique of traditional clinical approaches to meaning and trauma because it directly engages with the philosophical assumptions upon which these are built. His thought provides support for the sort of *context-centred* approach being developed in this book. In particular, his move away from a focus on the individual mind existing in relationship to an 'outside' world and towards an embedded notion of being-in-the-world, promotes a perspective in which contextual issues are not simply 'acting from the outside' on a series of reified psychological processes. His notion of 'worldliness' moves us away from scientific reductionism. Instead, existence in a world 'of significance' is primary and cannot be grasped or explained in an idiom of causal science. This works to contradict the fundamental tenets of positivism. Finally, Heidegger's account of human temporality, in which the future, past and present exist in a unified way helps us to avoid the difficulties encountered in the very concept of PTSD and highlighted by Allan Young (discussed in the last chapter).

In the next chapter I will explore the way in which Heidegger's thought was brought to bear directly on the fields of medicine and psychiatry through his long collaboration with Medard Boss, and in doing so I will tease out some further implications of this approach for our understanding of trauma.

Chapter 6
A Heideggerian approach to psychology and psychotherapy

Introduction

After the end of World War II, because of his earlier association with the Nazi party, Heidegger had to appear before a 'Denazification Commission' in Freiburg. He was forbidden to teach for three years, the ban lasting up to 1949. He was, however, allowed to keep his library and was granted an emeritus professorship by the University. In 1946 he received a letter from the Swiss psychiatrist, Medard Boss, who expressed an interest in applying the insights of *Being and Time* in his psychiatric work. Boss wrote later that he received 'an extremely warm response' from Heidegger. The two men met for the first time in Heidegger's hut in the Black Forest in 1947. This was the beginning of a long and productive friendship. According to Boss, Heidegger later revealed that to him that he (Heidegger) originally saw their involvement with one another as a means whereby 'his thinking would escape the confines of the philosopher's study and become of benefit to wider circles, in particular to a large number of suffering human beings' (Boss 1988a: 7).[1]

In this chapter I will examine the product of this collaboration. I will first point to some of the ways in which Heidegger's original account of Dasein was developed in the Zollikon seminars (see below) and then discuss aspects of Boss's Dasein-analytic psychotherapy. In the next chapter I will discuss Heidegger's approach to moods, and to the mood of anxiety in particular, as this relates directly to the question of trauma and loss of meaning.

Medard Boss and the Zollikon seminars

Boss was a psychiatrist who received psychiatric training from the two Bleulers (father and son) at the famous Burghölzhi hospital in Switzerland. He also had a training in psychoanalysis. He had begun his own analysis with Freud in 1925 and had continued it with Karen Horney in Berlin. He was also taught by Reich, Fenichel and Jones, amongst others, and participated for 10 years in a bi-weekly seminar with Carl Jung (Richardson 1993). In spite of this exposure to the major psychiatric and psychoanalytic thinkers of his time, Boss was dissatisfied with the prevailing accounts of human psychology and mental illness. He found Heidegger's account of Dasein in *Being and Time* extremely convincing. After reading this, he spent the rest of his life developing an approach to medicine and psychiatry based on Heidegger's thought. He received substantial support and encouragement from Heidegger himself in this endeavour. In the preface to the first edition of his 'magnum opus', *Existential Foundations of Medicine and Psychology*, Boss wrote that 'this work actually evolved under Heidegger's watchful eye. There is not one section of "philosophical" import which was denied his generous criticism' (Boss 1979: xxiii–xxiv).

At Boss's request Heidegger gave a series of seminars for Zurich-based medical doctors and psychiatrists between the years 1959 and 1969.[2] Although these seminars occurred many years after the publication of *Being and Time*, and in other writing of this time Heidegger had moved away from a central focus on Dasein, the major topics of discussion are the familiar themes of being-in-the-world and the existential structure of Dasein in terms of spatiality and temporality.[3] In addition, Heidegger discusses certain psychosomatic phenomena and generated an account of the bodily existence of Dasein that is not well developed in *Being and Time*. He also discussed, and severely criticized, Freudian psychoanalysis and distanced himself from the type of 'psychiatric daseinanalysis' being developed at that time by Binswanger. In this section I shall give an account of Heidegger's position on these issues, with supporting material from Boss. In the next section, I will briefly outline the main tenets of Boss's form of daseinanalysis.

'Bodyhood' and illness

In the seminars, Heidegger distinguished between the body as *Körper* and the body as *Leib*. The former refers to the physical body whose limit is the skin, the latter is the 'horizon' of the world for Dasein as being-in-the-world. Boss develops this approach to the body in a number of works. In *Existential Foundations of Medicine and Psychology* (English translation by Stephen Conway and Anne Cleaves) the word *Leib* is said to have the connotation of body as 'lived bodyliness'. The translators use the word 'bodyhood' in the text and give the dictionary definition of this as 'the quality of having a body or of *being body*'. Boss argues that scientific medicine has fundamentally misunderstood the nature of human bodyhood. By defining it in purely material terms as an object that can be measured and manipulated, science misses its specifically human dimension. He says:

> By positing the human body as some self-contained material thing, natural science disregards everything that is specifically human about human bodyhood. The natural scientific research method treats the body as it might treat works of art. Given a collection of Picasso paintings, for instance, this method would see only material objects whose length and breadth could be measured, whose weight could be determined, and whose substance could be analyzed chemically. All the resulting data lumped together would tell us nothing about what makes these paintings what they are; their character as works of art is not even touched by this approach.
>
> (Boss 1979: 100)

He makes the point that when a human being 'is existing' in the most characteristically human way it ceases to be aware of its bodyhood. Ironically, to be involved in a task whereby one puts one's 'body and soul' into it, is to be involved in such a way that one is not conscious of being a body at all. In spite of this, there is no aspect of human existence that is not bodily in some way. Being-in-the-world is to be a body. Even the most intellectual task involves what we have physically read or heard at some point. The point is that while Dasein is always embodied, simply regarding the human body as a thing fails to grasp the nature of this embodiment. Boss talks about human being as 'bodying forth' beyond the limits of the skin. When I perceive something, or point to something I am extending myself bodily beyond the reach of my fingertips. Just as there can be no independently existing time outside human temporality so too there is no such thing as a *human* body outside a human life. For Boss, echoing Heidegger in the quote above:

> The borders of my bodyhood coincide with those of my openness to the world. They are in fact at any given time identical, though they are always changing with the fluid expansion and contraction of my relationship to the world.
>
> (Boss 1979: 103)

In this interpretation of bodyhood, even the least gesture – a move of the hand, for example – can never be fully understood if the hand is simply regarded as a physical object made up of skin and bone and muscle. The human hand is so intimately related to being-in-the-world that it ceases to be a hand if this relationship is severed. A hand cannot exist except as a bodying-forth, an aspect of human engagement with the world. Thus a hand is only a hand because it is involved with a particular human existence. Likewise my organs of sensation: ears, eyes, touch owe their being to their involvement with an ongoing human openness to the world.[4] Thus bodyhood always presupposes a perceiving and acting existence, a human encounter with the world. Human existence 'bodies forth' through the different parts of our bodyhood. This means that bodyhood is 'phenomenologically secondary, though our senses tell us that it is primary' (Boss 1979: 105).

The meaning of this assertion becomes clearer in Boss's discussion of illness. This he defines as a state in which the potential to be fully human and free is undermined. With Heidegger, he argues that the fundamental existential 'traits' of human being are not 'so many bricks with which Da-sein is put together'. These traits are inseparable and all equally primary. Together they make up the structure of human being-in-the-world. Whenever one trait is disturbed, all the others are affected, and conversely, no matter how serious the illness, as long as the human is alive, these traits continue to exist, even if in potential only. He lists these fundamental traits, or Existentials, as:

> . . . the spatio-temporal character of *Da-sein*, its attunement, its bodyhood, its coexistence or being together with other people in a shared world, its openness and finally, the unfolding of inherent poten-tialities into existential freedom.
>
> (Boss 1979: 199)

There is also the 'ultimate existential trait of mortality'. These traits are what make human life human. Together they constitute Dasein as a 'clearing' in which the world comes to light. Illness involves impairment to one or more of these traits. Because of the presence of illness the human being is unable fully to actualize itself. As noted above, this does not mean that the trait is not present, for this would be to say that human life is not present. Rather, in illness the particular trait is seen to exist as blocked potential. For example, a child born without the use of its arms, because of prenatal thalidomide damage or perinatal injury to nerve fibres, has had its ability to 'body forth' in a relationship of greeting (by being unable to shake hands) reduced. In this way we see that it is because a specifically human being is present that a specific form of bodyhood impairment can come into being. Thus, human illness is dependent on human existence for its reality. The potential given to Dasein by its constitution in terms of the traits outlined above is what determines the nature of human illness. If we were not beings for whom communication is a part of our very make-up, then there would be no human illnesses characterized by a loss, or breakdown, of communication.[5] This is what Boss means when he says that 'bodyhood is phenomenologically secondary'. We can only build up a picture of bodily function and impairment from a prior understanding of what meaningful human reality is like. We cannot move in the other direction. Let us think of a painting by Picasso, and imagine that it has been damaged in a move from one gallery to another. The impact of the damage can only be judged by way of reference to the meaning of the painting as a whole. Loss of a certain amount of material from one corner of the painting might not render the painting as damaged as a loss from some other point on the canvas. The damage is *defined* by how the painting works as a meaningful whole. Boss uses the example of colour blindness. He makes the point that this condition is supposed to be clearly and primarily 'hereditary-organic'. However:

> If we want to understand what it really is, we will have to find out from the afflicted person exactly how his ability to relate himself through perception to what reveals itself to him in his world has been impaired. We will discover that he cannot respond to the meanings 'red' and 'green'. Yet the potentiality in understanding 'red' for what it is cannot be understood on the basis of any molecular structure. Like color blindness, all of the other so-called primarily organic-hereditary illnesses are by nature nothing more than deficiencies in the ability to carry out potential ways of being which are usually there for people.
>
> (Boss 1979: 201)

This discussion of bodyhood echoes the discussion of significance in the last chapter. We experience our world as, first and foremost, a world involving relationships of significance. We produce a scientific (in terms of physics and chemistry) account of that world only by stripping it of these relationships. The positivist and reductionist approach to the human world tries to move in the reverse direction, claiming along the way that the scientific world-view is actually primary. When it comes to the world of medicine, traditional approaches attempt to explain illness by 'working up' to 'subjective' human reality from the 'objective' descriptions of physics, chemistry, biology and (more recently) computer science. The 'phenomenological' account of illness developed by Heidegger and Boss attempts to reverse the direction of understanding, moving from lived human 'bodyhood' and being-in-the-world to an understanding of how certain phenomena limit the potential of this world.

Heidegger's critique of Freud

In the *Zollikon Seminars* Heidegger also developed a critique of Freudian psychoanalysis. He accused Freud of trying to force human being into a causal framework whose phenomena could be explained in terms of unconscious instincts and forces. Such unconscious elements were theoretical constructs, of which we could have no direct experience. The enterprise of phenomenology was very much to move in the opposite direction: to stick with, and never abandon, the phenomenon one sought to understand. He says:

> In the entire construct of Freud's libido theory . . . is there ever any room for 'man' (or human existence)? . . . Instinct [*Trieb*] . . . is always an attempt at explanation. However, the primary issue is never to provide an explanation, but rather to remain attentive to the *phenomenon* one seeks to explain – to what it is and how it is.
>
> (Heidegger, quoted in Dallmayr 1991: 214)

Attempts to explain human reality and behaviour through theories of instinct are always misconceived, because the human world can never be grasped through such a causal idiom. Heidegger also criticizes Freud's theory of repression. In this it is postulated that certain wishes, and other experiences, are so potentially distressing that they are banished from consciousness and stored instead in the unconscious. This theory is one of the fundamental cornerstones of psychoanalysis and reckoned by Freud and his followers to be one of his greatest 'discoveries'. The theory of repression has been widely used to explain such things as neurotic symptoms, the parapraxes, jokes and dreams. For Heidegger, this approach is mechanical and treats human reality on an ontic level, i.e. treats it as an object, among others in the world. If we accept that human being is ontological, according to Heidegger, then we need an approach that does justice to this fact. In the *Zollikon Seminars* he attempted to develop such an approach. In the last chapter we saw how Heidegger discussed human reality as a *Lichtung*, a clearing in which the world is brought to light. In place of repression, he proposed the 'intertwining of concealment and unconcealment, of clearing and veiling'. Dallmayr quotes him as follows:

> 'Freud's notion of repression,' we read, 'has to do with the hiding or stashing away of an idea or representation [*Vorstellung*].' By contrast, concealment (*Verbergung*) is 'not the antithesis to consciousness, but rather belongs to the clearing – a clearing which Freud did not grasp.'
>
> (Dallmayr 1991: 215)

Boss uses an example of a 'parapraxis' to illustrate the difference between the Freudian notion of repression and what is involved in the Heideggerian approach. A parapraxis involves some error in our everyday functioning. While most people regard such things as slips of the tongue and the forgetting of names as insignificant, for Freud these constituted the 'psychopathology of everyday life'. They come about because repressed desires seek to 'escape' from the unconscious mind, or because an unconscious wish blocks a consciously planned course of action. For example, if someone makes a slip of the tongue, this is interpreted by the psychoanalyst as meaning that he/she was unconsciously resisting what he/she consciously intended to say (Fenichel 1946: 312). Boss says that if, after spending an evening with a friend, he does not remember to take his umbrella, most people would say that he forgot it. However, a psychoanalyst might well interpret this as being caused by an unconscious wish to return to see the friend again, soon. The opportunity to do so has been created by the excuse to return for the umbrella. Boss says that this explanation is unconvincing as it makes no effort at understanding the forgetting of the umbrella as 'forgetting'. Instead it has made use of a hypothetical assumption that has nothing to do with the 'phenomenon under investigation'. A better account would involve staying with the notion of forgetting. Boss says that if this is taken to mean that the object is 'lost to the collection of objects in my world' then this is obviously not true. Boss still knows that he has an umbrella and knows what it looks like. The umbrella is still present in his world, although because he is engrossed in conversation with his friend, its presence becomes 'unthematic'. He says:

> My forgetting cannot be caused by the repression into an unconscious of my conception of the umbrella. In order to force something inward, I would need to have it in my grasp. Yet it is clear that while I am taking leave of my friend, I am with him, not with my umbrella. Thus I cannot possibly be occupied with a desire to forget it so I may visit him again. Such desire cannot be operating at that moment, consciously or unconsciously, because my whole being is occupied with my friend and with the topic of the evening's conversation. Here, forgetting is nothing more than the changing of a phenomenon's immediate, thematically considered presence in a human realm of openness to its nonimmediate and unthematic presence somewhere in the world.
>
> (Boss 1979: 117)

In this way, ideas, thoughts and desires may be 'neglected' or 'concealed' (Heidegger's term) or 'unthematically present' (Boss's term) but they are never 'put somewhere else'. There is, for the phenomenologist, an inherent contradiction in the very notion of a conscious–unconscious split. Boss quotes Kohli-Kunz on this subject. She argues that the concept of repression is really about self-deception. This is analogous to my deception of someone else. When I tell someone else a lie, I am aware of the truth, they remain unaware. When deceiver and deceived are, in fact, two different people there is no problem. When this is applied to one person there is a logical difficulty:

> In order to create the duality that was logically necessary to accommodate repression as self-deception, Freud took the integral selfhood of human existence, objectified it as a psychic apparatus, and split it into two pieces, the consciousness and the unconscious.
>
> (Kohli-Kunz, quoted in Boss 1979: 246)

Freud himself wrote:

> The term 'unconscious' refers to any psychic process whose existence we are forced to assume on the evidence of its outward effects but of which we know nothing directly. We stand in the same relation to this as to some psychic process in another person, except that here it is one of our own.
>
> (Freud, quoted in Boss 1979: 246)

If this is the case, and conscious and unconscious are as one person is to another, then there must be some 'agent' acting to decide which repressed material will be allowed to become conscious. Freud calls this agent the 'censor'. But this must have the ability to review, deliberate and decide. In other words, it must be conscious, in some way. We end up with a censor that is an 'unconscious consciousness'. Kohli-Kunz argues that the only way out is to reject Freud's 'reification of human being-in-the-world' and his 'compartmentalization' of the psyche. While she still opts to use the word 'repression', this is clearly not Freudian repression but something very similar to the Heidegger/Boss approach. She says that, in the phenomenological outlook, Dasein is 'integral, indivisible being-in-the-world', and in this 'repression' becomes a:

> . . . very specific mode of human conduct towards something that is encountered, i.e., a refusal to admit the address and urgent appeal of encountered beings, a looking away from them, a fleeing from them. This is flight from the concrete beings actually perceived in a world . . . Repression, then, is anything but a mechanical shuttling of representation between compartments of a psyche. In repression, what is repressed is not set aside. Rather, it becomes increasingly obtrusive. The urgency of the appeal of what the closed and narrowed being-in-the-world cannot admit becomes more and more intense.
>
> (Kohli-Kunz, quoted in Boss 1979: 246–47)

Thus, for Heidegger, and those phenomenologically-orientated psychiatrists who followed him, Freud's work represented a continuation of the

Cartesian project. Mental substance, split off from bodily substance, was to be investigated in the same mechanical idiom used by physical science. Heidegger spoke about the 'fatal distinction between conscious and unconscious' (see Richardson 1993: 54). However, Freud was not the only psychiatrist criticized in the course of the *Zollikon Seminars*. Heidegger also made a number of negative assertions about the form of phenomenology and 'psychiatric daseinanalysis' being developed by Ludwig Binswanger.

Heidegger on Binswanger

Like Boss, Binswanger was a Swiss psychiatrist who had studied with Eugen Bleuler and Carl Jung, who introduced him to Freud in 1907. In 1911, Binswanger became the chief medical director at Bellevue Sanatorium in Kreuzlingen. Although he remained a friend of Freud's until the latter's death in 1939, in the 1920s and 1930s he gradually moved away from a Freudian perspective and, under the influence of Husserl and Heidegger, developed an existentialist approach. Although Binswanger called his work 'daseinanalysis' and cited Heidegger as his main philosophical influence, in the *Zollikon Seminars* Heidegger claimed that Binswanger had seriously misunderstood much of his work.[6] Heidegger accuses Binswanger of paying insufficient regard to the ontological–ontic difference. Because of this there is a tendency for him to misunderstand the fundamental nature of Dasein as a 'clearing'. Instead Dasein becomes a 'subject', or an 'ego', in either case a 'thing' amongst other things. For Heidegger, this is Cartesianism. Any analysis of Dasein worthy of the name must start with Dasein's ontological dimension, its relation to 'being-ness as a whole'. This does not happen in Binswanger's 'psychiatric daseinanalysis'. Heidegger says:

> So little can this relation to being-ness be omitted from the leading and all-important determination of Dasein that by overlooking precisely this relation [as happens in the 'psychiatric daseinanalysis'] we are prevented from ever thinking adequately of Dasein as Dasein. The understanding-of-Being is not a determination relevant only to the thematic of fundamental ontology but is *the* fundamental determination of Dasein as such. An *Analysis* of Dasein therefore that omits this relation to Being-ness as such which is essential in the understanding-of-Being is not an Analysis of *Dasein*.
>
> (Heidegger 1988: 85)

Heidegger argues that Binswanger completely misunderstands the notion of care (*Sorge*) as developed in *Being and Time*. For Heidegger, Dasein is always in a relationship of care with its world. It is only because such care is a fundamental part of the existential make-up of Dasein that we live in a world that has significance for us. Care thus refers, in *Being and Time*, to the way that Dasein is actually structured. It should not be regarded as just one psychological disposition among others. Heidegger remarks that Binswanger had selected the notion of 'being-in-the-world' but had interpreted it in an empirical-contextual sense. This is an important observation because Binswanger says that his whole approach is based on the notion of being-in-the-world.

In the next chapter I shall present Heidegger's approach to anxiety and the loss of meaning and I shall link this with the question of trauma. I will conclude this section by mentioning Heidegger's brief remarks about 'stress' in the *Zollikon Seminars*. These are of interest, given our concern with trauma and post-traumatic stress disorder (PTSD) in this book. Commenting on a psychiatric report dealing with the subject, he contrasts his approach to that of behaviourism, which conceptualizes stress as a stimulus, impacting upon the human being from outside. Instead, Heidegger conceives of stress as something which 'lays claim' to Dasein's care (*Beanspruchung*). This claim cannot be understood in terms of a stimulus-response but only in terms of a situated being-in-the-world. Demands on Dasein come about because of its basic 'thrownness' in the world. He says:

> Only on the basis of the correlation of thrownness and understanding
> via language can Dasein be addressed by beings; the possibility of such
> an address, in turn, is the condition of the possibility of a demand or
> claim – whether this takes the form of stress or of relief from stress.

> (Heidegger, quoted in Dallmayr 1991: 222)

Boss also writes about stress and notes the ambiguity involved in any event or experience. One circumstance will be a source of stress for one person, not for another. This, he notes, is a cause of some frustration for those using a natural science approach. Science tries to render every 'object' of study into a form whereby it can be 'calculated' in some way. He says:

> . . . not out of regard for the object of study itself, immense effort is
> expended in the natural sciences, including medicine, to get rid of the
> inherent ambiguity of phenomena and reduce them to a condition of
> unambiguous calculability.

> (Boss 1979: 207)

However, he observes that there is simply no such thing as an unambiguous or 'self-contained' stimulus. Thus for the phenomenologist, stress exists for human beings because human being is 'openness' to the world and thus can be the object of demands from that world. Many of these demands are experienced as ambiguous. This analysis resonates with the analysis of trauma presented in Chapter 4. We encountered Allan Young's writing in which there is an inherent ambiguity about the relationship between contextual issues, stressful events and their sequelae. In fact, no event can be objectively described as traumatic. The way in which any event is experienced will always depend on the context and the individual history of the person involved. We noted that the *DSM III* of 1980 had assumed that certain events could be inherently traumatic. Clinical experience led to the abandonment of this assumption in later versions of the *DSM* (see also Chapter 3).

Daseinanalysis

We have noted above the gap between Heidegger and Binswanger. In this section I shall briefly describe the essential aspects of the form of dasein-analysis developed by Boss and his colleagues. Boss maintains that there are two aspects to daseinanalysis. First there is daseinanalysis as ontology. This incorporates a way of understanding human reality that challenges traditional medical, psychiatric and philosophical accounts of human being. This aspect is closely based on the writings of Heidegger, in particular on *Being and Time*, and some of the major themes of this understanding were introduced in the last chapter and in the section above. In this section I wish to concentrate on the second aspect: dasein-analysis as a specific form of psychotherapy. While sympathetic to the general thrust of Boss's thought it will become clear that I am not convinced that his daseinanalysis is an adequate response to the implications of Heidegger's thought. It remains a form of psychotherapy, focused on an individual patient. To my mind, if we accept Heidegger's account of being-in-the-world we are challenged to understand and to respond to madness and distress in terms of contexts. This cannot happen within the confines of a psychotherapy framework.

Daseinanalysis and psychoanalysis

Boss says that daseinanalysis involves an approach to therapy:

> . . . which is concerned with freeing individuals to fulfil their own-most possibilities for being with things and with other human beings. Although all serious psychotherapies are concerned with this very thing, with liberating individuals from the suffering and constriction which prevents them from being themselves, only daseinanalysis has a philo-sophical understanding which comprehends this as the goal and purpose in the first place.
>
> (Boss 1988b: 62)

While Boss and his followers were quite clear that their approach was very different to other forms of psychotherapy, they have not sought to establish an 'official' account of what this approach involves in practice. Their assumption seems to be that if the therapist can properly grasp the philosophy involved, then the therapeutic techniques follow on from this. Indeed, while Boss was deeply critical of Freud's theory, there is no evidence that he had any great misgivings about his (Freud's) therapeutic techniques. In his book *Psychoanalysis and Daseinanalysis* (published originally in 1957), Boss wrote that he remained impressed with the power of 'Freud's unsurpassed practical recommendations' (Boss 1963: 285). Indeed, Boss saw his project as involving an attempt to 'restore the original meaning of Freud's actual, immediate, concrete and most brilliant observations' (Boss 1963: 59).

One of Boss's followers was Gion Condrau. He became Director of the training institution founded by Boss in Zurich – the *Daseinanalytic Institute for Psychotherapy and Psychosomatics*. In a seminar published in 1988, Condrau indicated that in daseinanalysis patients lie on a couch, as in conventional psychoanalysis. They are also invited to 'free associate'. This is 'the basic ground rule' of psychoanalysis, introduced by Freud. The patient is instructed to say anything that comes into his/her mind. Condrau says that whereas in Freudian analysis this technique is used in order to allow repressed wishes and other material to emerge from the patient's unconscious, in daseinanalysis it is used in order 'to give the patient as much freedom as possible' (Condrau 1988: 118). Similarly, daseinanalysis makes use of the other Freudian therapeutic technique – dream interpretation.

Dream interpretation in daseinanalysis

Boss actually wrote two books on dream interpretation. The first was published in 1953. This was translated into English and published in 1958 as *The Analysis of Dreams*. In this Boss set out to 'pave the way for the direct study of the dream phenomenon itself, by removing all the disguises and schemata of mental constructs of contemporary dream theories' (Boss 1958: 10).

While he again gives credit to Freud for drawing attention to the meaningful nature of dreams he goes on to criticize him for his 'scientific' and 'objective' account. He is particularly critical of Freud's positing of the manifest dream as a secondary phenomenon and his turn instead to the latent, or hidden, meaning of the dream as the primary target of interpretation. For Boss, the manifest dream is what should be approached in therapy. In addition, it should not be presumed that the elements of the manifest dream 'stand' for or symbolize something else. His approach is to 'stay with the phenomena' which are presented in the reported dream. In the seminar mentioned above, Gion Condrau gives an example of a dream that was discussed at a meeting of analysts from different schools. The dream was one that had been reported by a young woman to one of the participants. The woman had dreamed that, while sleeping one night, the window in her room flew open and a piece of wood was hurled into the room. She dreamed that she 'woke up' and found the wood on the floor. This then became a snake that proceeded to slide underneath the woman's bedclothes. At this point she 'actually' awoke in a state of fear. Condrau reports that for the Freudians the snake represented 'phallic anxiety', whereas for the Jungians the snake was a symbol of unconscious spiritual forces. For Jung, himself, the snake was always a symbol of individuation. In the Jungian framework this would be interpreted as an 'archetypical' dream indicating that the dreamer was in an important phase of personal growth. Condrau says: 'Well, as daseinanalysts, we would first argue that this dream snake is not a symbol at all. A snake is a snake, even in the dream.' However, this does not mean that nothing further can be said about the dream:

> A snake is an animal, an instinct-bound living creature; and we would say that the person who dreamt this sees something, recognizes something, is related to something about this kind of creatureliness. Also, we see that something opens up to this dreamer in the dream, not only did the window open, but the dreamer 'opened,' that is, she woke up, she opened up into waking while still dreaming. Just the fact that she sleeps and then wakes up in the dream, means that she is seeing something, opening up to something, perhaps for the first time.
>
> (Condrau 1988: 121)

Nineteen years after his first book on dream analysis, Boss (1977) published another work on the subject: *I dreamt last night . . . .* In this he gives 115 pages of dream analyses and again exhorts the reader to stay with the manifest dream and not postulate unconscious forces that give rise to the content. Rather, the dream is understood as an experience of concentrated attention and emotion. In this experience, one's relationships to other people and to the things of the world are laid open, sometimes in 'uncomfortable closeness'.

The 'attitude' of the therapist in daseinanalysis

A very good example of the daseinanalytic approach to dream interpretation is provided by the American therapist Erik Craig (1988b). He takes Freud's famous 'dream of Irma's injection' that is the central dream in *The Interpretation of Dreams*, and subjects it to the daseinanalytic approach.

By concentrating on the actual elements of the reported dream Craig is able to develop an interesting (and for me convincing!) account of Freud's 'existential' situation at the time of the dream (the summer of 1895). However, I do not wish to focus on Craig's reading of the Irma dream as such. Instead I want to point to his account of 'anticipatory care' that is said to be characteristic of the daseinanalytic approach to therapy. To grasp the meaning of this concept will require a return to the text of *Being and Time*.

In *Being and Time* Heidegger spoke about the nature of Dasein's 'Being-with' others as *Fürsorge*. The translators of the work note that there is no good English language translation but they opt for the word 'solicitude'. They remark that although this is more literally translated as 'caring-for', this

> . . . has the connotation of 'being fond of', which we do not want here; 'personal care' suggests personal hygiene; 'personal concern' suggests one's personal business or affairs. 'Fürsorge' is rather the kind of care which we find in 'prenatal care' or 'taking care of the children' or even the kind of care which is administered by welfare agencies.
>
> (Macquarrie and Robinson, footnote in Heidegger 1962: 157)

Heidegger goes on to point out that, in a negative direction, solicitude can mean something approaching, but never in fact fully equating, indifference. However, it can also be a 'positive' encountering of others. There are two 'extreme possibilities' of such positive solicitude. On the one hand we can 'intervene' in someone's life (*einspringende Fürsorge*). Solicitude can, as it were,

> . . . take away 'care' from the Other and put itself in his position in concern: it can *leap in* for him. This kind of solicitude takes over for the Other that with which he is to concern himself. The Other is thus thrown out of his own position; he steps back so that afterwards, when the matter has been attended to, he can either take it over as something finished and at his disposal, or disburden himself of it completely. In such solicitude the Other can become dominated and dependent, even if this domination is a tacit one and remains hidden from him.
>
> (Heidegger 1962: 158)

The German word *einspringen* is often used in situations where one person 'steps in' for another. It has the connotation of taking over responsibility for the other person's life and actions. Craig suggests that it is the form of care often seen in medicine and even in therapy. On the other hand, solicitude can mean a way of relating to the other in which one:

> . . . does not so much leap in for the other as *leap ahead* of him
> [*vorausspringt*] in his existentiell potentiality-for-Being, not in order to
> take away his 'care' but rather to give it back to him authentically as such
> for the first time. This kind of solicitude pertains essentially to authentic
> care – that is, to the existence of the Other, not to a '*what*' with which he
> is concerned; it helps the Other to become transparent to himself *in* his
> care and to become *free for* it.
>
>   (Heidegger 1962: 158–59)

Heidegger says that, for the most part in everyday life, we relate to one
another in a way that is a mixture of these two extremes:

> Everyday Being-with-another maintains itself between the two extremes
> of positive solicitude – that which leaps in and dominates, and that
> which leaps forth and liberates [vorspringend-befreiend]. It brings
> numerous mixed forms to maturity . . .
>
>   (Heidegger 1962: 159)

Craig (following Boss) argues that this second type of solicitude, this form
of 'anticipatory care', was exactly what Freud was seeking to achieve in the
practice of psychoanalysis. However, his orientation towards medical
science often pulled him in the other direction, and undermined this.
Craig maintains that the manifest content of the dream of Irma's injection
is centred on a tension between these two forms of care. Initially, in the
'dream plot', the Freud character is in a mood of openness and receptivity;
later, with the appearance of Irma, his persona becomes medical, analytic
and intrusive, more concerned about the views of his peers than about
Irma's own account of herself. Craig gives the following interpretation,
based on his phenomenological interpretation of the dream:

> First we must remember that Freud's sudden 'retreat' to medicine and
> biology was in part an act of professional conscientiousness, a shoul-
> dering of the models and attitudes of physicianly care which he had
> been taught and in which he so deeply believed. We must also
> remember, however, that at this very juncture of his life, Freud was in
> the midst of a revolutionary paradigmatic change and consequently was
> on his way to seeing that there was more to this physicianly care than the
> giving and receiving of 'solutions' and 'injections'. Increasingly he was
> becoming aware of the significance of the uniquely human and
> 'meaning-full' dimensions of psychological care including especially the
> significance of the human relationship between doctors and patients.
>
>   (Craig 1988b: 213)

At numerous points in his work Boss argues that Heidegger's description
of a non-dominating form of solicitude is actually the ideal mode of care

for the psychotherapist. He suggests that this is, in fact, what Freud recommended as 'the best possible therapeutic attitude' (Boss 1963: 74).

The limitations of daseinanalysis

While my presentation of the literature on daseinanalysis has been far from comprehensive, it does emerge that this form of therapy does not present or develop any new techniques of its own. Daseinanalysis is revealed, in the writings of Boss and his followers, to be a sort of 'philosophically sophisticated psychoanalysis'. Patients come, on an individual basis, to see a therapist. They lie on the couch, free associate and offer dreams for interpretation. The therapist adopts a position of 'anticipatory care' and helps the patient face the challenges of his/her life. As mentioned above, its goal is an expansion of individual freedom. In a number of places, Boss argues that the most important question that the therapist can ask his/her patient is not 'Why?', but 'Why not?' While theoretically, Boss, with the help of Heidegger, put considerable 'distance' between himself and Freud, practically, in the therapeutic arena there is not a great deal of difference between the two. Eric Craig himself says:

> Beyond the radical phenomenological rethinking of the essentials of psychotherapy, including its unique structure and meaning as well as its most ubiquitous and characteristic phenomena, daseinanalysis has added little that is novel to the actual conduct and practice of the craft.
>
> (Craig 1988a: 16)

One has the sense of being promised much more. The Heideggerian understanding of human reality is so profoundly different to the philosophical tradition that underscores Freudian psychoanalysis that one expects the implications for psychiatry to be equally profound. Instead we are guided down a path that leads into the familiar territory of individual psychotherapy. It must be said of Boss that in an afterword to his major work *Existential Foundations of Medicine and Psychology* he spoke briefly about the 'Foundations of a *Da-sein*-based Social Psychology and Social Preventive Medicine in Modern Industrial Society'. In this piece he echoes Heidegger's reflections about the nature of technological civilization (which I shall examine in a later chapter). However, Boss's thoughts are very sketchy and his proposals are weak. Essentially he seems to argue that in modern industrial society there is more time for recreation than ever before, and because this is the only time in which human beings have the potential to relate to one another outside the world of capitalist alienation, recreation is an area worthy of the interest of daseinanalytical psychologists and psychiatrists. More guidance than this we simply do not get. Technological rationality is so pervasive that there appears to be little hope that we can take steps to move beyond. In fact, those of us who live in the Western world can really only 'wait':

> We may assume that the break through the technological framework of modern industrial society into a genuine freedom in relation to this technology will not be done first by the West. It is rather to be hoped for from the peoples of the Far East . . . (whose) being-in-the-world . . . is shaped always, continually, and decisively by a traditional relationship with the world that is astonishingly close to the vision of European phenomenology just now unfolding.
>
> (Boss 1979: 296)

It would appear that Boss's background as a psychiatrist influenced strongly by psychoanalysis led him to adapt Heidegger's thought to the type of human encounter set up by psychoanalysis. Daseinanalysis involves a rethinking of psychoanalysis rather than an opening up of a genuinely alternative approach within psychiatry.

Given the Heideggerian insights about the nature of Dasein's being-in-the-world and about the importance of Dasein's pre-ontological understanding of its world one could have expected that a psychiatry based on Heidegger's thought would have moved in a direction away from individual psychotherapeutics and more towards a focus on the relationship between mental illness and the social and cultural world. While I have great sympathy with Boss's striking respect for the cultures of India, China and Japan, the above comments are obviously inadequate in terms of helping the development of a form of social psychiatry that is not ultimately grounded in a Cartesian philosophy. As mentioned in the introduction, one of my aims in this book is to explore how Heideggerian ideas can help us to substantially rethink the whole world of distress, madness, psychiatry and healing. In Section 3 we shall return to the question of what a non-Cartesian psychiatry might look like.

Summary

In this chapter I reviewed the collaboration between Heidegger and the psychiatrist Medard Boss in the years after World War Two. I discussed their approach to 'bodyhood', the phenomenology of illness and their critique of Freudian theory. I noted Heidegger's objections to the form of 'daseinanalysis' developed by Binswanger. I gave an account of Boss's form of daseinanalysis that is essentially a form of psychoanalysis influenced by Heideggerian thought. At the end of the chapter I expressed my disappointment with this work. In the next chapter I shall examine Heidegger's understanding of anxiety and connect this with the current discourse on trauma. This will then allow me to present an alternative to current cognitivist accounts of the 'loss of meaning' often described after trauma.

Chapter 7
Meaning, anxiety and ontology

Introduction

In Chapter 5, I discussed Heidegger's approach to the understanding of human being. I attempted to show how this approach differed from the traditional framework of psychology and in particular from the cognitivist orientation that, as we have seen, dominates current thinking in the area of trauma. Heidegger offers us an approach which insists on the embedded nature of human reality, a reality in which the cultural and temporal are not merely additional factors which can be added to an independent psychology but are in fact a priori dimensions of our reality which allow for a psychological world in the first place.

In this chapter I shall return to the question of meaning and its loss and explore Heidegger's phenomenological approach to this. Guided by the ontological/ontic difference explored in Chapters 1 and 5, I want to suggest that there is an *ontological* dimension to the question of meaning.

Heidegger's understanding of mood

The structure of Being-in

Being and Time is essentially an analysis of the nature of Dasein's being-in-the-world. Dasein, as an entity, is always ontological, so Heidegger calls his exploration of Dasein a 'fundamental ontology' (1962: 170). Because this exploration does not take for granted the usual starting point of psychology, i.e. a subjective realm relating to an outside objective world, Heidegger's account of human experience is radically different from traditional accounts. Thus his examination of such things as our sense of self, moods, cognitions and death is of a very different nature from those found in mainstream psychology.

He says that while being-in-the-world is a 'unitary phenomenon' this does not prevent it from being analysed in terms of the 'several constitutive items in its structure' (1962: 78). First, he analyses what it is to be 'in-the-world' and defines his notion of 'worldhood'. We saw in Chapter 5 how for Heidegger the human world is always primarily a place full of significance and we explored some of the implications of this in relation to scientific reductionism. After the question of 'where', Heidegger takes up the question of 'who'. He says he wants to look at the 'entity which in every case has Being-in-the-world as the way in which it is. Here we are seeking that which one inquires into when one asks the question "Who?"' (Heidegger 1962: 79).

In this analysis he directs his attention mainly to the fact that we exist in a social world: our being, our identity and self-understanding, is always bound up with other people. This is Dasein as 'being-with' (*Mitsein*). Third, he analyses the notion of being-in (*In-sein*). We have already seen how Heidegger argues that Dasein's being-in cannot be thought of as one entity being in another, as is the case when we say, for example, the water is in the glass. We have already encountered his presentation of Dasein as a 'clearing', what Heidegger terms a *Lichtung* (see Chapter 5). Thus Dasein is always orientated in one way or another. Being-in is never a neutral, unaffected, uninvolved illumination, but is, as it were, focused in a particular way. I argued that our opening up of a world is dependent on our embodiment (having a body) and our existence in a social world. These elements combine so that we are able to encounter a world that is meaningful. Heidegger says that there are two aspects of this opening up: understanding (*Verstehen*) and mood or orientation (*Befindlichkeit*). These are not present as distinct but are always experienced in a unitary way. Thus, according to Heidegger, human being is always situated, and as such always already has a position of understanding and is always in some way in a 'mood' or 'state-of-mind' (see next section). We never encounter the world in a 'neutral' way. As we are concerned with Heidegger's concept of *Angst* which is a 'state-of-mind' we shall proceed by first giving an account of his concept of *Befindlichkeit*.

Befindlichkeit

As with the term *Dasein*, there is considerable dispute with regard to the translation of the term *Befindlichkeit* into English. Macquarrie and Robinson indicate that the literal translation would be something like 'the state in which one may be found'. They point out the connection with the common German expression '*Wie befinden Sie sich?*' which literally means 'How are you?' or 'How are you feeling?' They reluctantly use the expression 'state-of-mind', while pointing out its limitations. However, Dreyfus argues that this is completely unacceptable. He says:

> To translate this term we certainly cannot use the translators' term, 'state-of-mind', which suggests, at least to philosophers, *a mental state*, a determinate condition of an isolable, occurrent subject. Heidegger is at pains to show that the sense we have of how things are going is precisely *not* a private mental state.
>
> (Dreyfus 1991: 168)

What we need, according to Dreyfus, is an English word that conveys a sense of 'being found in a situation where things and options already matter'. He opts for the word 'affectedness'. McCall also condemns Macquarrie and Robinson's translation, suggesting that we use something like 'the sense of one's actual situation'. *Befindlichkeit* refers, he says, to an 'orienting attitude of the individual toward his actual situation' (McCall 1983: 77–78). This seems too personalistic and open to the same objection raised by Dreyfus. Gendlin discusses the term *Befindlichkeit* at some length and argues that in grappling with this concept we go to the 'core' of Heidegger's philosophy. According to Gendlin:

> '*Sich befinden*' (finding oneself) . . . has three allusions: The reflexivity of finding oneself; feeling; and being situated. All three are caught in the ordinary phrase, 'How are you?'. That refers to how you feel but also to how things are going for you and what sort of situation you find yourself.
>
> (Gendlin 1988: 44)

He says that Heidegger's coinage of the term *Befindlichkeit* is 'clumsy' and there is simply no English language equivalent which transmits the sense of 'how-you-are-ness'. For the most part I will use the translator's term, 'state-of-mind', or the original *Befindlichkeit* in the following discussion but I am aware of the limitations of this approach. At times I shall resort to the word 'mood'. With *Befindlichkeit*, Heidegger is clearly referring to something like the familiar concept of 'mood' or 'feeling' or even the term used in clinical psychiatry – 'affect'. However, his point is that behind these everyday notions there also lies an ontological dimension. Moods are not simply 'things' which can be analysed and dissected unproblematically. They are part of the way in which a world is revealed. They allow us to be 'attuned' to the world.

Being in a mood or state-of-mind is one of the fundamental ways that Dasein is aware of its being-in-the-world. Thus, state-of-mind is one of the ways in which Dasein discloses being. The implication is that state-of-mind, or its everyday mode, 'mood', should not be thought of as something internal and mentalistic. There is always a background or public dimension:

> A mood assails us. It comes neither from 'outside' nor from 'inside', but arises out of Being-in-the-world, as a way of such Being . . .
> Having a mood is not related to the psychical in the first instance, and is not in itself an inner condition which then reaches forth in an enigmatical way and puts its mark on Things and persons.
>
> (Heidegger 1962: 176)

Gendlin argues:

> Whereas feeling is usually thought of as something inward, Heidegger's concept refers to something both inward and outward, but before a split between inside and outside has been made.
> We are always situated, in situations, in the world, in a context, living in a certain way *with others*, trying to achieve this and that.
>
> (Gendlin 1988: 44)

The point is that our usual understanding of mood or feeling as something private and internal is false to the true nature of our experience. This echoes the discussion at the beginning of Chapter 5. Our moods are not 'inside' and separate from an 'outside' world. Our moods are part of the process through which a world is brought to light. Our moods have a social dimension and, as we shall see, are always culturally embedded, just as our understandings of the world are. Only in the context of our background cultural orientation to feeling can we have individual feeling and mood.[1]

Anxiety

By now the reader will not be expecting a 'conventional' clinical approach to the question of anxiety! For Heidegger, anxiety (*angst*) is not a patho-logical mood. It is something 'built into' our constitution as human beings. As a form of *Befindlichkeit* it is part of the process through which we encounter the world. Before discussing anxiety Heidegger presents an analysis of the related mood of fear. He says that there are three ways in which we can consider the phenomenon of fear:

1. That in the face of which we are afraid: the 'fearsome'. This is the thing in the world that threatens us and brings about the state of fear.
2. Fearing as such. This is the actual mood that allows something to show up as being a threat. Fear is thus something that discloses the world to

us. It is a good example of a mode of state-of-mind which is one of the equiprimordial aspects of being-in, one way in which Dasein as being-in 'illuminates' the world:

> We do not first ascertain a future evil (malum futurum) and then fear it. But neither does fearing first take note of what is drawing close; it discovers it beforehand in its fearsomeness. And in fearing, fear can then look at the fearsome explicitly, and 'make it clear' to itself. Circumspection sees the fearsome because it has fear as its state-of-mind. Fearing, as a slumbering possibility of Being-in-the-world in a state-of-mind (we call this possibility 'fearfulness' ('Furchtsamkeit')), has already disclosed the world, in that out of it something like the fearsome may come close.
>
> (Heidegger 1962: 180)

Imagine an encounter with a storm. To experience the wind and rain in their true awesomeness I must be able to have some degree of fear in relation to the weather. I must be able to fear, to feel threatened. Without the mood of fear being available to me I will not be able to perceive the danger of the weather and thus its power and potential. My fear, even if only in the background, is essential to my understanding and appreciation of the nature of the weather. It is part of the way in which the world of weather is disclosed to me.

3. That which fear fears about, Dasein itself, is what is threatened in situations of fear. This can relate to things other than simply parts of one's body. Dasein can be threatened by attacks on its projects. Fear can be with regard to the things that Dasein is concerned with and fear can be in the form of 'fearing for' when one is afraid on another's behalf.

Based on this analysis of fear we can say that, according to Heidegger's account, the structure of moods consists of (a) the before-what of moods, (b) the mood itself and (c) the about-what of moods (Smith 1981: 221). Armed with this structure Heidegger is able to approach the question of anxiety.[2]

Heidegger discusses anxiety at some length in *Being and Time*. This makes sense if we remember that the overall aim of this work is to do 'fundamental ontology', to use an analysis of Dasein to open up the question of being in a new way. In writing about anxiety Heidegger is not just presenting us with an example of a particular state-of-mind. I have already noted Heidegger's use of the term *Sorge* (care). This represents the ontological structure of Dasein. This term should not be taken to have the English language connotations of love or affection. In *Being and Time* it indicates the fact that Dasein is always occupied, in some way, with the entities it encounters in the world. Human beings always 'care' about the world and what they are doing, even if this is only out of narrow self-interest. Things always matter to us. As being-in-the-world, Dasein simply cannot avoid being involved with and dealing with the world. Heidegger explores the existential phenomenon of anxiety because it reveals, as nothing else can, this 'care-structure' of Dasein. Just as a breakdown in the workings of a piece of equipment can reveal the nature of the equipment and how it actually functions[3], in analysing anxiety Heidegger is attempting to reveal the nature of Dasein and its world. In the state-of-mind of anxiety Dasein is brought to a halt and forced to examine its true situation as being-in-the-world. For the most part Dasein exists not as a free entity facing its own destiny and its own possibilities but rather as one in the midst of the many, in the midst of the 'They' (*Das Man*), taking its directions from the crowd. The experience of anxiety, however, causes Dasein to feel dislocated with regard to *Das Man* and thus precipitates a fundamental examination of its own predicament. Thus, in *Being and Time*, and in the essay 'What is Metaphysics?' (in Heidegger 1993), anxiety is presented not simply as an unpleasant mood but as a state-of-mind which can serve the function of revealing to Dasein its true predicament.

Heidegger begins by contrasting anxiety and fear and makes the point that the two are often thought of as referring to the same thing:

> We are not entirely unprepared for the analysis of anxiety. Of course it still remains obscure how this is connected ontologically with fear. Obviously these are kindred phenomena. This is betokened by the fact that for the most part they have not been distinguished from one another: that which is fear, gets designated as 'anxiety', while that which has the character of anxiety, gets called 'fear'.
>
> (Heidegger 1962: 230)

However, on the basis of his analysis of fear Heidegger is able convincingly to assert a difference. Most crucially is the question of what it is that anxiety is anxious about. As fear relates to the fearsome, what is it that anxiety is about?

> What is the difference phenomenally between that in the face of which anxiety is anxious (*sich ängstet*) and that in the face of which fear is afraid? That in the face of which one has anxiety is not an entity within-the-world.
>
> (Heidegger 1962: 230–31)

> *That in the face of which one has anxiety (das Wovor der Angst) is Being-in-the-world as such.*
>
> (Heidegger 1962: 230)

In fear, Dasein is threatened by some entity in the world. In anxiety it is the question of being itself that has become threatening. It is the question of how anything makes sense at all. For what happens in anxiety is that Dasein comes face to face with a terrifying feeling that the background connections that make sense of and order the entities of the world have receded. Anxiety is anxious because of an absence, not a presence:

> That in the face of which one has anxiety is characterized by the fact that what threatens is *nowhere*.
>
> (Heidegger 1962: 231)

Heidegger's separation of the mood of anxiety from that of fear is uncontentious and echoed by many writers on the subject.

For example, Kurt Goldstein speaks about anxiety as attacking us 'from the rear'. Writing in the late 1930s, Goldstein says that while in the situation of fear we are aware of ourselves and well aware of the object of our fear: 'Does not anxiety consist intrinsically of that inability to know from whence the danger threatens?' (Goldstein 1939: 292).

What Heidegger describes as anxiety is a profound sense of the constructed nature of the world and the connections of the entities within it. In anxiety we look at the order of the world as if from outside. The meanings, values, roles of our lives appear as devoid of any ultimate grounding. In Chapter 1 I used an analogy from the world of chess. In anxiety it is as if the playing board in a game of chess was taken away: the pieces are still there but their relatedness has disappeared. Their positions in relation to one another become arbitrary and lack significance; thus moving them becomes meaningless. In anxiety, the world, in the sense of a structured whole, withdraws from us. The entities within the world: the people, the places, the things, the projects are still there in situ as before, but their sense has vanished and with it any orientation towards a future or any sense of purpose. Everything appears strange and disconnected. Heidegger uses the term *Unheimlich* which is usually translated as 'uncanny' but means more literally, 'unhomelike':

> As we have said earlier, a state-of-mind makes manifest 'how one is'. In anxiety one feels *'uncanny'*. Here the peculiar indefiniteness of that which Dasein finds itself alongside in anxiety, comes proximally to expression: The 'nothing and nowhere'. But here 'uncanniness' also means 'not-being-at-home' (das Nicht-zuhause-sein).
>
> (Heidegger 1962: 233)

It is this experience of *Unheimlichkeit* which is at the heart of the mood of anxiety. In *Being and Time* anxiety is the mood that reveals the groundlessness of the world and Dasein's being-in-the-world. Dreyfus says:

> Anxiety is thus the disclosure accompanying a Dasein's preontological sense that it is not the source of the meanings it uses to understand itself; that the public world makes no intrinsic sense for it and would go on whether that particular Dasein existed or not. In anxiety Dasein discovers that it has no meaning or content of its own; nothing individualizes it but its empty thrownness.
>
> (Dreyfus 1991: 180)

In the essay 'What is Metaphysics?' this disclosive function of anxiety is also discussed. Anxiety is seen as revealing the nothingness at the heart of Being. Metaphysics is, in essence, concerned with the question of being and nothingness. In Heidegger's framework neither of these terms has a concrete empirical reference. Thus we cannot approach an understanding of nothingness by way of a simple definition. Nothingness is neither a positive entity nor is it simply the negation of such an entity, it is in fact 'more original than the "not" and negation'. In other words nothingness 'is the source of (logical) negation, not the other way around'. Thus negation depends on Dasein having a prior access to an experience of nothingness. In anxiety, according to Heidegger, Dasein has such access:

> We cannot say what it is before which one feels ill at ease. As a whole it is so for one. All things and we ourselves sink into indifference. This, however, not in the sense of mere disappearance. Rather, in this very receding things turn toward us. The receding of beings as a whole that closes in on us in anxiety oppresses us. We can get no hold on things. In the slipping away of beings only this 'no hold on things' comes over us and remains.
> Anxiety reveals the nothing.
>
> (Heidegger 1993: 101)

Thus the question of anxiety becomes a central focus of metaphysics. In this essay anxiety is presented as something ever present but out of view. It is a most fundamental mood but ordinarily we live our lives oblivious to its presence because we are absorbed in the everyday world. However, we need to cease our flight from anxiety, according to Heidegger, if we are to engage in any real metaphysical enquiry. In anxiety there is disclosure of the lack of any foundational grounding for the meaningfulness of the world. We realize that the world has no meaning outside of Dasein and thus Dasein itself is the ground. Dasein is the 'groundless ground' and has to provide a meaning that will not otherwise be given. As well as disclosing something essential about the nature of Dasein, anxiety also discloses something about the nature of the world. As Joseph Fell summarizes:

> The blanking out of everyday significance does not leave us with nothing at all; beings remain, but now as strange, stripped of their ordinary familiarity. Abruptly, they stand out like sore thumbs, all by themselves, independent of any grounding context. Not nothing, they *are* – but for no evident reason or purpose, without 'whence or whither'. This is the routinely concealed human experience of the disclosure of sheer givenness, sheer contingency, the disclosure of naked 'that-being' . . . Anxiety is thus the beginning and a basis of all specifically human ontic experience and ontological understanding.
>
> (Fell 1992: 69)

Thus the anxiety discussed in *Being and Time* and in 'What is Metaphysics?' cannot be conceived as a symptom, a sign of breakdown. It is clearly something built into the nature of Dasein and its being-in-the-world. It is, in fact, an 'originary' experience out of which various other human experiences flow. Even though it is a profoundly uncomfortable experience and we usually are at pains to avoid it, it is never really absent from our lives. Heidegger says:

> . . . original anxiety in existence is usually repressed. Anxiety is there. It is only sleeping. Its breath quivers perpetually through Dasein.
>
> (Heidegger 1993: 106)

Anxiety and death

In the first section of Division II of *Being and Time* Heidegger reiterates the aim of the entire work: it is to investigate the meaning of being in general, and since the meaning of being is disclosed by Dasein the ultimate clarification of the meaning of being demands an equally ultimate (or primordial) interpretation of Dasein. What is required is an approach to Dasein that can grasp it as a 'whole'. He goes on to point out that his analysis in Division I is less than complete because it has failed to reveal both the totality and the authenticity of Dasein. He says:

> One thing has become unmistakeable: *our existential analysis of Dasein up till now cannot lay claim to primordiality*. Its fore-having never included more than the *inauthentic* Being of Dasein, and of Dasein as *less* than a *whole* (*als unganzes*). If the Interpretation of Dasein's Being is to become primordial, as a foundation for working out the basic question of ontology, then it must first have brought to light existentially the being of Dasein in its possibilities of *authenticity* and *totality*.
>
> (Heidegger 1962: 276)

We shall raise certain problems with Heidegger's notion of authenticity in the next chapter. For now I simply want to explain how this connects with his approach to anxiety. Essentially, Heidegger is arguing that because, for the most part, Dasein is bound up in a social world where meanings and beliefs are simply given, the individual does not have to face up to his/herself and our lonely place in the universe. In fact, a great deal of social life is about allowing us to avoid any real encounter with this reality. This allows us to live our lives in a sort of inauthenticity. Facing anxiety with 'resoluteness' is about moving beyond this to a more authentic mode of existence. Division II of *Being and Time* is an attempt to move the analysis of our condition in this direction. It is through an analysis of death that Heidegger proceeds, as it is only in its being-toward-death that Dasein is revealed in its totality and it is only through the lucid acceptance of one's death that Dasein moves towards authenticity. Death both totalizes and individualizes Dasein. As long as Dasein is still alive it continues to choose its possibilities, it is always 'ahead-of-itself':

> It is essential to the basic constitution of Dasein that there is *constantly something still to be settled*.
>
> (Heidegger 1962: 236)

There is, he says, always a 'lack of totality'. Death provides this sense of totality to Dasein's existence. At the same time death provides each one of us with the one and only experience which is uniquely ours and in facing death we have the opportunity to define ourselves as somehow distinct from the 'They' (*Das Man*), to define for ourselves the meaning of our lives and to achieve a sense of authenticity which otherwise would be always only partial.

While death allows Dasein its possibilities of totality and authenticity, the cost is the ever-present reality of anxiety:

> But the state-of-mind which can hold open the utter and constant threat to itself arising from Dasein's ownmost individualized Being, is anxiety. In this state-of-mind, Dasein finds itself face to face with the 'nothing' of the possible impossibility of its existence.
>
> (Heidegger 1962: 310)

In anxiety we are brought into a relationship with our own death. As death is something that cannot be confined to a particular moment or period of time, and yet can materialize at any moment, it is essentially and profoundly indefinite. The indefiniteness of the threat of death undermines our connections with the public world, for it demonstrates, as nothing else can, the fragility and unreliability of this world. None of the meanings, the connections, the narratives given to us by our social world can protect us from death. As discussed above, the essential quality of the

mood of anxiety is this sense of disconnection, of groundlessness. Thus in
Division II Heidegger links together anxiety and death in a very clear way:

> Being-towards-death is essentially anxiety.
>
> (Heidegger 1962: 310)

In summary, in the early work of Heidegger anxiety is presented in
the following ways:

1. Anxiety is not a symptom of illness or disease but a mood available and
   present to all. On the other hand what Heidegger is describing is not
   just an unease that emerges in the course of philosophical reflection.
   He presents us with a phenomenological understanding of a state-of-
   mind which is extremely painful. This is why, for the most part, we
   attempt to avoid it. However, anxiety never completely disappears from
   a human life and is always present, even if only as a potentiality. In
   certain situations anxiety can become part of a person's daily life and
   can be a reason for a presentation to psychiatry.
2. Unlike fear, anxiety is not 'about' any entity in the world. Anxiety is
   experienced in relation to being as a whole. It is an experience of the
   nothingness at the heart of being. Fear is actually the mood most often
   encountered in those conditions labelled by psychiatry as 'anxiety
   disorders'. However, moods such as fear, depression and alienation are
   often accompanied by the sort of anxiety defined by Heidegger.
3. Anxiety can be a privileged revealing experience of our essential nullity
   and rootlessness. In facing anxiety we have the potential to move to an
   'authentic' mode of being.
4. There is an intimate relationship between anxiety and death. Anxiety is
   the state-of-mind in which we have an experience of our own mortality.
5. Anxiety is best characterized as a sense of being 'ill at ease'. In it, the
   world is experienced as profoundly strange. We feel 'not at home'
   (*Unheimlich*) in the world.

In what remains of this chapter I will relate this analysis to the question of
trauma. I will show how the cognitivist and phenomenological
(Heideggerian) approaches to meaning open up different ways of framing
the problems and possible solutions.

Janoff-Bulman's 'new psychology of trauma' revisited

As we saw in Chapter 3 a number of clinicians and researchers have
attempted to conceptualize the ways in which traumatic events have their

impact. I drew attention to the fact that at the heart of the concept of PTSD lies the symptom complex of intrusion-avoidance phenomena. These symptoms appear to be associated with the victim's search for meaning, and cognitive theories that aim to grasp this search for meaning have come to dominate current theoretical work on PTSD.[4] A recurrent theme in this context is the idea that extremely frightening events have the effect of shattering the background assumptions of the individual with regard to him/herself and with regard to the order of the outside world. As we saw in Chapter 2, cognitive psychology involves an account of human reality in which each of us is said to develop a set of assumptions (also called schemas or scripts) about our worlds and ourselves. In the cognitive approach the meaningfulness of our lives is dependent on these assumptions. Like most other psychological theories, cognitivism does not recognize the sort of ontological/ontic difference described by Heidegger. Cognitivism encounters the issue of meaning on an ontic level. It assumes that, like other aspects of psychology, it can be investigated by an empirical, fact-seeking approach. We shall return to the difference between hermeneutics and cognitivism on the question of meaning below.

In Chapter 3 we saw how, in her book *Shattered Assumptions: Towards a New Psychology of Trauma* (1992), Ronnie Janoff-Bulman, following the cognitivist tradition, argues that there is a universal and definable structure to human psychology. She argues that trauma has the effect of disturbing our basic assumptions about ourselves and the meaningfulness of the world in which we live. The victim of trauma is left with both a fear of threats from the environment which remind him/her of the trauma and also a sense of 'disillusionment' due to a shattering of his/her assumptive framework. There are obvious incompatibilities between Janoff-Bulman's account of human reality and that of Heidegger. We shall examine these below. However there are strong resonances between her account of post-traumatic sequelae and Heidegger's account of fear and anxiety. Janoff-Bulman's distinction between terror and disillusionment is similar in many ways to Heidegger's distinction between fear and anxiety, even though at times she uses the term anxiety as being synonymous with fear.[5] Terror, which she equates with fear and anxiety, relates to external threats, whereas disillusionment relates to the 'inner world'. This echoes Heidegger's proposal that fear is produced by a threat from some entity in the world whereas anxiety is generated from a concern with the background meaningfulness of the world. Janoff-Bulman says:

> Fear and anxiety are dominant early responses to overwhelming life events; represented physiologically as arousal and cognitively as the perception of threat, these emotions can persist months or even years

after the traumatic event. Yet a very different psychological reaction
typically co-exists with the fear and anxiety, and this is the experience of
profound disillusionment, a response that often outlasts a victim's fear
and anxiety. Victims' inner worlds are shattered, and they see their prior
assumptions for what they are – illusions.

(Janoff-Bulman 1992: 70)

Just as Heidegger described anxiety as a profound sense of disconnection,
many people who have been through something very frightening describe
being 'cut-off' in some way from the world. The experience of very frightening events can have the effect of shattering any sense of living in an
orderly world that has inherent structures of meaning and order.

People describe a feeling of being set adrift from the rest of the world,
of being completely on their own in a way which is beyond ordinary
loneliness. The feeling of trust in the world, both human and natural,
which is essential to ordinary life, has been broken apart and people
describe living in a meaningless void, desperately seeking their old sense
of order and meaning. The combat veteran Tim O'Brien describes how for
the common soldier in the midst of war:

> There is no clarity. Everything swirls. The old rules are no longer
> binding; the old truths are no longer true . . . The vapours suck you in.
> You can't tell where you are, or why you're there, and the only certainty
> is overwhelming ambiguity. In war you lose your sense of the definite,
> hence your sense of the truth itself, and therefore it's safe to say that in a
> true war story nothing is ever absolutely true.
>
> (O'Brien 1990: 88)

Post-traumatic anxiety also involves a profound realization of the self's
fragility. Just as Heidegger related anxiety and death, the literature on
post-traumatic reactions provides numerous accounts of how post-
traumatic anxiety is connected to a sense of one's imminent death. Robert
Lifton, after interviewing 75 survivors of the atomic bomb in Hiroshima 17
years after the event, described them as exhibiting what he called a 'death
imprint'. This reaction was also reported in other groups such as survivors
of the concentration camps and survivors of natural disasters. Lifton
argued that the 'death imprint' is the key to understanding post-traumatic
reactions: 'what needs (also) to be emphasized is the survivor's having
experienced a *jarring awareness of the fact of death* . . . he has been
disturbingly confronted with his own mortality' (Lifton 1967: 481).

The encounter with death serves to emphasize the fragility of the self:
we can no longer operate with any sense of invulnerability. There is
nothing we can do to avoid death. A traumatic event brings this realization
home with considerable force. Thus post-traumatic anxiety combines a

penetrating sense of the ultimate meaninglessness of the world and a paralysing sense of the self's fragility in the face of death. As we have already seen, Heidegger's account of anxiety emphasizes very similar themes.

Thus, Janoff-Bulman's description of post-traumatic disillusionment resonates strongly with Heidegger's account of anxiety. Both accounts are of a phenomenon which is to be distinguished from fear of an outside threat. Both accounts describe a phenomenon that is essentially a mood of dislocation associated with a profound sense of a lack of meaning and order. Both accounts stress the relationship between this phenomenon and the apprehension of death. My suggestion is that traumatic experiences can have the effect of awakening the mood of anxiety in individuals. According to the Heidegger of *Being and Time*, however, this mood is 'already there' in every human being and not something brought about *de novo* by the trauma. Rather, trauma can have the effect of *revealing* the anxiety that is a built-in dimension of human being.

Broken meanings, broken worlds

Ontological understanding involves an exploration of being, an exploration of the fact that a meaningful world is open to us. This is something very different to science. If I am correct, and the mood-state described by Heidegger in terms of anxiety is of a similar nature, in descriptive and experiential terms at least, to the mood-state described by Western psychology as occurring after trauma, then it follows that an ontological exploration of post-traumatic anxiety is a path worth taking. Current ways of approaching trauma, and particularly cognitive approaches, clearly operate on an ontic level and treat the question of meaningfulness in the same way that they treat other aspects of psychology, i.e. as 'something' to be analysed. My suggestion is that this approach is inadequate because the meaningfulness of the world, or in Heideggerian terms the meaning of being, cannot be grasped by this type of analysis. This issue demands ontological understanding.

We saw in the last chapter how Medard Boss approached an understanding of illness. He argued that we cannot build up a picture of illness from a description of a particular lesion in itself. Illness involves a limitation of the Dasein's ability to be itself, to be fully open to the world as only Dasein can be. To understand this, we need, as a first step, a full understanding of the meaningful nature of this human world. The phenomenological approach to illness moves from a description of everyday human reality to lesion in order to understand fully the limitations imposed on that reality by the lesion in question. If post-traumatic anxiety is characterized by a withdrawal of meaning, then we need to understand how a meaningful world *is present for us in the first place*. What is it that withdraws from us in this state?

If Heidegger's account of Dasein is found to be convincing, then science (whether biological or psychological), will have great difficulty accounting for this meaningfulness. Following the Heideggerian analysis of human reality developed in Chapter 5, and examples of the phenomenological approach 'in action' in the last chapter, we are now in a position to explore the question of meaning from a phenomenological position. Following Heidegger, to do this properly we must avoid any of the starting assumptions of traditional psychology. In particular, we must deal with experience as we find it before it has been shaped by any sort of theory. We begin with the fact that we find ourselves, first and foremost, in the world and with the world in us. We are not separate, and cannot be separated from, our worlds. They are fundamental dimensions of ourselves. As we have already seen, Heidegger goes to great pains to overcome the Cartesian assumptions which have become built into our understandings of ourselves, indeed have become built into the language we commonly use to describe ourselves. These are assumptions to the effect that mind stands outside world and is related to it by means of representations. The central Cartesian problematic concerned the question of how we can ever know the world 'outside' us. Heidegger does not answer this because his starting point is not a situation where subject and world are separate in the first place, and the one stands in a position of 'knowing' the other. As Stephen Mulhall puts it:

> . . . [knowing] is therefore doubly inapplicable as a model for the ontological relation between subject and world. First, because knowing is a possible mode of Dasein's Being, which is Being-in-the-world; knowing therefore must be understood in terms of, and cannot found, Being-in-the-world. Second, because knowing is a relation in which Dasein can stand towards a given state of affairs, not towards the world as such; Dasein can know (or doubt) that a given chair is comfortable or that a particular lake is deep, but it cannot know that the world exists. As Wittgenstein might have put it, we are not of the *opinion* that there is a world: this is not a hypothesis based on evidence that might turn out to be strong, weak or non-existent.
>
> (Mulhall 1996: 96)

For Heidegger, for the most part, we do not relate to our world by having sets of schemas stored in our minds concerning the world. Likewise, the meaning of the world is not something located, or 'encoded' in Bolton and Hill's account, inside individual minds. Rather, the meaning of the world, and of ourselves as part of that world, lies in the background intelligibility generated by the everyday shared beliefs, rituals and practices through which we as embodied beings engage with that world. It is also dependent on the fact of our embodiment (see Taylor's discussion of how embodiment provides a 'built-in' orientation towards the world in Chapter 5). These elements have the effect of allowing the entities of the world to show up as meaningful. Entities only have meaning against a background that renders them intelligible. While our conscious beliefs are important, Heidegger, like Wittgenstein, puts his emphasis on this background, which cannot be grasped as a set of beliefs at all. In fact, according to Wittgenstein, the practices that are the basic elements of our forms of life are overwhelmingly complicated and he warns against attempts to systematize the 'bustle of life'. In his *Remarks on the Philosophy of Psychology, Volume II* he says:

> The background is the bustle of life. And our concept points to something within this bustle.
>   And it is the very concept 'bustle' that brings about this indefiniteness. For a bustle comes about only through constant repetition. And there is no definite starting point for 'constant repetition'.
>
> (Wittgenstein 1980: 108)

While Heidegger is involved in an attempt to characterize the common-sense background and illuminate its structure, he is firmly against the idea that it can be grasped as any sort of set of concepts or schemas. According to Heidegger we have a 'pre-understanding' of the world that is neither conscious, nor unconscious. Dreyfus uses a number of examples to illustrate what could be involved in such a 'pre-understanding'. In his book *What Computers Still Can't Do: A Critique of Artificial Reason* (1994) he points to the difficulties that proponents of artificial intelligence have with the question of background knowledge. While programs can be written which allow computers to 'play' rule based games like chess, programmers have had serious difficulties trying to develop programs which can grasp basic aspects of the human environment. They have a particular problem with the equipment we use in our everyday lives, equipment that makes sense only in relation to embodied 'cultured' creatures like ourselves. Dreyfus says:

> No piece of equipment makes sense by itself. The physical object which is a chair can be defined in isolation as a collection of atoms, or of wood or metal components, but such a description will not enable us to pick out chairs. What makes an object a *chair* is its function, and what makes possible its role as equipment for sitting is its place in a total practical context. This presupposes certain facts about human beings (fatigue,

the way the body bends), and a network of other culturally determined
equipment (tables, floors, lamps), and skills (eating, writing, going to
conferences, giving lectures, etc). Chairs would not be equipment for
sitting if our knees bent backwards like those of flamingos, or if we had
no tables as in traditional Japan or the Australian bush.

(Dreyfus 1994: 37)

As living social beings, humans have a 'pre-understanding' which allows
them to live in a world that makes sense. Chairs relate to tables, floors and
lamps. In turn, how something is revealed as a table is dependent on its
connections with other entities and with us as the users of such things.
The web of meaningful connections that provide the background context
in which something shows up as a chair reaches out in all directions. It is
not something that can be grasped as a set of concepts, rules or schemas.
Because of this computer programmers have so far failed to crack this
'frame' problem. Another example of our 'pre-understanding' is 'distance-
standing practices':

> People in different cultures stand different distances from an intimate, a
> friend, a stranger. Furthermore, the distances vary when these people
> are chatting, doing business, or engaging in courtship. Each culture,
> including our own, embodies an incredibly subtle shared pattern of
> social distancing. Yet no one explicitly taught this pattern to each of us.
> Our parents could not possibly have consciously instructed us in it since
> they do not know the pattern any more than we do. We do not even
> know we have such know-how until we go to another culture and find,
> for example that in North Africa strangers seem to be oppressively close
> while in Scandinavia friends seem to stand too far away.

(Dreyfus 1994: 294)

We become uneasy in such situations and try different stances until we feel
more comfortable. As Dreyfus remarks, it is presumably through some
responses like this in early life that we learned about distance in the first
place. However, for the vast majority of us, this learning was not through
the acquisition of concepts concerning standing and relationships:

> As a skill or *savoir faire* it is not something like a set of rules that could
> be made explicit. Yet it embodies rudiments of an understanding of
> what it is to be a human being – hints of how important body contact is,
> and the relative importance of intimacy and independence.

(Dreyfus 1993: 294–95)

As Dreyfus points out, human practices like distance-standing involve
particular orientations towards the world. In this way our deepest values
are actually embodied in our practices. Another source of examples of

how an understanding, and a way of life, can be contained non-cognitively in our practices is the work of Erving Goffman. In his book *Relations in Public* (1971) Goffman analyses the phenomenon of 'civil indifference'. This occurs in modern societies when strangers pass each other on the street. It involves an implicit understanding about the correct way to encounter one another. One person acknowledges the other through a controlled glance. This indicates a degree of respect but is non-intrusive. The person then averts their gaze to show that there is no threat intended. The other person does the same. This encounter incorporates a tacit understanding of the nature of human reality and the relationship between individuals. It is a ritual embedded in the urban world of modernity and involves 'modern' ways of understanding the world and other people. In many traditional societies where there is a more clear-cut difference between who is a 'familiar' and who is a 'stranger' people generally do not encounter each other through such rituals of 'civil indifference'. They may completely avoid one another or else stare in a way that would be perceived as threatening in a modern context. Giddens notes that such rituals of everyday life, involving trust and tact, are more than merely ways of protecting one's self-esteem and that of others. Rather, in so far as they involve the very substance of everyday encounters with one another, 'they touch on the most basic aspects of ontological security' (Giddens 1991: 47).

The intelligibility of our worlds, their meaningfulness, is thus not something held as a set of schemas in an individual mind. The sense and order of our worlds are aspects that simply cannot be grasped, or formalized as a set of beliefs or rules or programmes. Dreyfus says that:

> Sense is precisely what is left out in all formalization. Sense, for Heidegger, in opposition to Husserl, is the structure of the general background that can never be fully objectified but can only be gradually and incompletely revealed by circular hermeneutic inquiry.
>
> (Dreyfus 1991: 222)

For the cognitivists, ruptured meanings occur inside individual minds. For Heidegger, because the inside-outside distinction is false and because meaning resides in our background practices, the breakdown of meaning involves this background. From a phenomenological point of view, loss of meaning occurs in a broken world, not a broken mind. Trauma has an ontological dimension because it can have the effect of bringing the intelligibility of the world into question. Post-traumatic anxiety is thus a state of Dasein in which the meaningfulness of life itself, and the situation of Dasein within life have been rendered fragile.

Because intelligibility and meaningfulness are social phenomena, derived from the practices of our everyday lives, the social world is not seen as something impacting on the post-traumatic state from 'outside'. Conceiving the social dimension of trauma in terms of 'social factors' acting as 'buffers' of one sort or another simply does not do justice to the lived reality of the survivor. If trauma is about broken meanings, then it is a social phenomenon through and through. In his writing, the psychiatrist Derek Summerfield, whose work was quoted in Chapter 4, draws attention to the importance of a socio-cultural dimension in modern conflicts. For example:

> Guatemalan Indians, hunted by 'low intensity' warfare, felt that their collective body had been wounded, one which included the ants, trees, earth, domestic animals and human beings gathered across generations. Mayan origin myths are linked to land and maize. To them the burning of crops by the army was not just an attack on their physical resources, but on the symbol which most fully represented the Mayan collective identity, the people of the maize. When they talked about 'sadness' they meant something experienced not just by humans but also by these other interconnected elements which had been violated. When you touched the earth you could feel its sadness, and you could taste it in the water. To them all this was genocide.
>
> (Summerfield 1998: 17)

In building their models of post-traumatic reactions, cognitivist researchers begin by positing some psychological process that is presented as the essential element of the reaction. They work with a model of an individual mind reacting to a specific event or series of events. They add to this ideas about pre-existing personality traits and cognitive schemas. To this are added ideas about the social environment. In other words, they theorize 'from the inside out'. In contrast, the phenomeno-logical approach 'moves in the other direction'. In this, the first step in understanding the impact of an event or series of events, on an individual or community, is the generation of an account of the social world that existed before and after the events. From this one moves to understand the meaningful world of any particular individual. Psychology cannot be divorced from an understanding of background context. While concepts and beliefs form part of this context, it is primarily constituted by our embodied, practical, human encounter with the universe. This can be illuminated but not comprehensively defined and grasped in a scientific idiom.

As a result of this analysis I believe that the (Heideggerian) phenome-nological account of meaning and intelligibility is better able to account for the importance of social and cultural environment in relation to trauma than that built on the Cartesian assumptions discussed in Chapter 2. The way in which one's world is meaningful and ordered will determine the way in which one experiences and reacts to any particular event. It will also determine what forms of help will be appropriate. In addition, Heidegger's approach to time and causality, discussed in Chapter 5, presents a fundamentally different picture of how individuals experience the events of their lives, compared to the traditional understanding embodied in the concept of PTSD. We have seen how this question of causality has brought about certain problems for the traditional framework. These problems simply do not arise within a Heideggerian phenomenology because all experiences are understood to occur within a horizon that encompasses past, present and future together. In this, my reaction to a terrifying event *always* happens in these three dimensions. Debates about whether my reaction was caused by the traumatic event or instead caused the event to be retrospectively highlighted (and thus the 'target' of my intrusive-avoidance symptoms) are seen, in the light of the Heideggerian account of human temporality, to be misconceived and not open to clear resolution.

In spite of these positive 'gains' from a phenomenological account of trauma, in the next chapter I shall point to certain difficulties that emerge from this account. At the centre of my concerns is Heidegger's own account of his project in *Being and Time*. In this work he operated with the assumption that there could be a 'fundamental ontology'. In other words, he appears to have believed that it would be possible to give an account of Dasein in universal terms. While he was opposed to any 'psychological universalism' (the positing of mental processes which were universal and which could be investigated scientifically), nevertheless he appears to have assumed that he was, in fact, exploring the structures of all human experience.[6] In his account of human reality in *Being and Time* anxiety plays a key role. In the next chapter I shall discuss how, according to the Heidegger of Division II of this work, it was only through the experience of anxiety that Dasein could become authentic. In *Being and Time* anxiety is always close at hand and, as we have seen above, is related to the fact of human mortality. While loss of meaning and intelligibility may well be universal human reactions, I shall argue in Section III against this assumption that anxiety plays the same role in every culture. I shall argue that in some cultures anxiety (as a state-of-mind characterized by a sense of dislocation and 'homelessness') is more 'close at hand' than in others. This will have important implications for the cross-cultural under-standing of trauma.

I also noted at the end of the last chapter my 'disappointment' with the limited therapeutic horizon opened up by daseinanalysis as developed by Boss and Heidegger. If post-traumatic anxiety involves the withdrawal of meaningfulness and order, and if these are given by the background practical way of life in which we live, then helping people who have been traumatized requires an effort to rebuild this way of life. Individual psychotherapy will make little sense to people, like the Mayan Indians described by Summerfield above, who have lost a way of life.

Summary

This chapter has moved between philosophy and psychology, between phenomenology and cognitivism. I have attempted to develop an understanding of 'loss of meaning' from a phenomenological point of view. This required an outlining of Heidegger's account of anxiety as presented in *Being and Time*. I then connected this with Janoff-Bulman's account of 'shattered assumptions' as an example of a cognitivist approach to the same issue. Using Heidegger, I argued that there is an ontological dimension to post-traumatic anxiety which cannot be grasped through the framework of an 'ontic' science such as cognitive psychology. Having presented the case for a hermeneutic approach to the issue of trauma, at the end of this chapter I pointed to some questions concerning the universal validity of Heidegger's account of anxiety. This is to raise some of the tensions that were identified in the introduction. In Section III these tensions will be explored further.

Chapter 8
Authenticity in question

Rethinking the place of anxiety

A number of commentators have drawn attention to a change in direction in Heidegger's thought in the 1930s. This has been compared with the substantial change in the philosophy of Wittgenstein that occurred after the *Tractatus*. The change in Heidegger's philosophy has been called his *Kehre*, or 'turning'. In this chapter, I will not dwell at length on the nature of Heidegger's *Kehre*, but will focus on the relationships between technology and nihilism in the later works. In Section III, I shall argue that anxiety (as discussed in the last chapter) is something that has an association with modernity and, more particularly, the shift to postmodernity. I want to make the case for a 'hermeneutic' appropriation of the insights of *Being and Time* in which we drop the 'universalist' understanding of anxiety as a revelatory mood at the heart of every Dasein.

Most commentators are now agreed that Heidegger's *Kehre* was more apparent than real. Essentially, it would appear that Heidegger moved on to explore different themes and away from the central focus on Dasein that characterized *Being and Time*.[1] Heidegger, himself, was willing to speak about a 'Heidegger I' who preceded this turning and a 'Heidegger II' who came after, but rejected any strong sense of a separation in the end. He says:

> . . . only by way of what [Heidegger] I has thought does one gain access to what is to-be-thought by [Heidegger] II. But the thought of [Heidegger] I becomes possible only if it is contained in [Heidegger] II.
>
> (Heidegger's preface in Richardson 1963: xxii)

All of Heidegger's thought has focused on the question of being. In *Being and Time* and other works from the same period he sought being through an analysis of Dasein: the being for whom being is an issue. Existentialist interpretations of *Being and Time* have tended to equate the question of being with questions about the projects of individualized Dasein. From the 1930s onwards Heidegger positions himself firmly against humanism. In his 'Letter on Humanism' (in Heidegger 1993: 217–65), written after the war, he specifically reacts against what he would regard as subjectivist approaches to phenomenology such as those of Sartre.[2]

However, a number of commentators have pointed to a tension within *Being and Time*, a tension between what I will loosely call the 'existentialist' and the 'hermeneutic' aspects of the work. This becomes most apparent in relation to the role of anxiety and the question of authentic and inauthentic ways of being. In *Being and Time* Heidegger is centrally concerned to investigate Dasein's way of being. However:

> Ontically, of course, Dasein is not only close to us – even that which is closest: we *are* it, each of us, we ourselves. In spite of this, or rather for just this reason, it is ontologically that which is farthest.
>
> (Heidegger 1962: 36)

In other words, there are aspects of our being that are so 'close to us' that we cannot 'see' them in our normal gaze. These aspects involve the 'foundations' of our lives and actions. In our daily lives we do not have to pay attention to these foundations, we simply take them for granted. In fact, we usually forget about them altogether. Heidegger argues that all our actions and behaviours are premised upon an 'already existing' interpretation of the world, what he calls our 'preontological understanding of being'. This is given to us by the culture in which we emerge as any particular embodied human being. Thus the culture in which we find ourselves provides us with a preconscious orientation towards the world. As we saw in the last chapter, this is not something we can stand apart from and examine because it structures our very ways of examining in the first place. As we saw in Chapter 5, Heidegger uses the term 'being-in-the-world' in an attempt to get beyond a notion of the human being as something separate from its world. He says:

> Dasein is never 'primarily' a being which is, so to speak, free from being-in, but which sometimes has the inclination to take up a 'relationship' toward the world. Taking up relationships toward the world is possible only *because* Dasein, as being-in-the-world, is as it is.
>
> (Heidegger 1962: 84)

Our worlds are always in us, as we are in our worlds. Thus our understanding of ourselves is always already structured for us. We cannot hope to develop an understanding of ourselves that is free from, or outside, the various possibilities thrown up by the culture in which we live, or by the cultures we have access to.

This is most clearly seen in relation to language. The words we use to understand ourselves are always 'common words', in the sense that they are always shared by the community in which we live.[3] In *Being and Time*, Heidegger uses the term *Das Man* to indicate the world of our everyday social involvement. This is the they-world. Dreyfus (1991) translates the term *Das Man* simply as 'the one'. It refers to the social world in which we normally live our lives. Dreyfus argues that there is a major internal contradiction in Heidegger's approach to this everyday social world. He says:

> Heidegger is influenced by Kierkegaard and Dilthey, both of whom had a great deal to say about the importance of the social world. But, whereas Dilthey emphasized the positive function of social phenomena, which he called the 'objectifications of life,' Kierkegaard focused on the negative effects of conformism and banality of what he called 'the public'. Heidegger takes up and extends the Diltheyan insight that intelligibility and truth arise only in the context of public, historical practices, but he is also deeply influenced by the Kierkegaardian view that 'the truth is never in the crowd'.
>
> (Dreyfus 1991: 143)

Although Dasein is always being-in-the-world (including the social world), Heidegger (perhaps following Kierkegaard) describes Dasein's everyday involvement in *Das Man* as 'fallenness'. He describes Dasein's 'fallen' involvement with the world as indicating a '*fleeing* of Dasein in the face of itself' (Heidegger 1962: 229). The result is that Dasein's existence, as existence in the mode of *Das Man*, is inauthentic. There is thus a normative element to Heidegger's account of Dasein as being-in-the-world. It would appear that while Dasein always exists with a 'preontological understanding' of the world, something that Dasein receives from the world of *Das Man*, nevertheless Dasein possesses the possibility of moving beyond this. This possibility is given, as we saw in Chapter 7, in the state of anxiety. In anxiety, Dasein experiences the world and all its meanings as contingent, without any ultimate grounding. In this state it is brought before itself as being, itself, the only ground. This is a painful and desperate moment and Dasein, normally, attempts to flee. In anxiety, Dasein is, so to speak, truly alone. Heidegger says:

> Anxiety thus takes away from Dasein the possibility of understanding itself, as it falls, in terms of the 'world' and the way things have been publicly interpreted. Anxiety throws Dasein back upon that which it is anxious about – its authentic potentiality-for-Being-in-the-world. Anxiety

individualizes Dasein for its ownmost Being-in-the-world, which as
something that understands, projects itself essentially upon possibilities.

(Heidegger 1962: 232)

There would thus appear to be a contradiction in Heidegger's account,
two incompatible accounts of inauthenticity. Dreyfus calls these the structural and motivational accounts. On the one hand, Dasein is involved in
the everyday social world because of structural necessity. It simply *is*
being-in-the-world. On the other hand, Dasein 'actively' flees into this
world to escape from the pain of anxiety. The latter account contains the
implication that Dasein could potentially change its position and move
away from its inauthentic participation in the world of *Das Man*. By
contrast the former account seems to undermine the very possibility of
such authenticity. The motivational account of inauthenticity is developed,
at length, in Division II of *Being and Time*. Heidegger further extends the
idea that it is Dasein's response to anxiety that determines whether it
becomes authentic or not. Dreyfus argues that Heidegger was involved in
an unsuccessful attempt to 'secularize' Kierkegaard's interpretation of the
Christian doctrine of the fall. For Kierkegaard, our distraction by the
practices of the everyday world constituted sinfulness. In Heidegger's
work this becomes fallenness. However, according to Dreyfus:

> Heidegger's attempted secularization runs into a double contradiction;
> inauthenticity becomes both inevitable and incomprehensible. On the
> one hand, if one holds that falling as absorption is motivated by fleeing,
> i.e., that absorption is a way of covering up Dasein's nullity, then, since
> absorption is essential to Dasein as being-in-the-world, Dasein becomes
> essentially inauthentic. On the other hand, if facing the truth about itself
> leads Dasein to equanimity, appropriate action, and unshakable joy,
> resoluteness is so rewarding that, once one is authentic, falling back into
> inauthenticity becomes incomprehensible.
>
> (Dreyfus 1991: 334)

At the heart of this contradiction lies Heidegger's indebtedness to both the
hermeneutic philosophy of Dilthey and the existentialist philosophy of
Kierkegaard. Dreyfus makes a case in favour of the former approach and
argues for a 'Wittgensteinian interpretation of being-in-the-world in terms
of shared background practices' (1991: 144). However, existentialists can
find in *Being and Time* strong support for a philosophy of life that emphasizes the importance of individual freedom and choice. In the later works
Heidegger left these tensions behind. The important point for our
discussion is that this analysis has clarified, to some extent at least, the
problematic position of anxiety, in *Being and Time*. As I wish to use
Heidegger's thought to help orientate an approach to the relationship

between meaning and trauma and, in particular, cultural aspects of this relationship, I want to shed the *universalist* existentialist dimension while holding on to the hermeneutic insights.[4] If Dreyfus is correct, and Heidegger's universalist presentation of anxiety and inauthenticity, is a secularized version of a (Kierkegaardian) Christian narrative then I feel justified in doing this. The Christian orientation to the world carries its own ontology and cannot be used to account for the realities of other, non-Christian and post-Christian cultures. In essence, I wish to hold on to Heidegger's depiction of anxiety as a state-of-mind in which the meaningfulness of the world withdraws from us, but leave behind his idea that this arises in the same way, and serves the same function, in all cultures.

I believe that this move is supported by textual evidence from Heidegger himself. *Being and Time* was published in 1927. In a lecture course given in 1929–30, and published first in an English translation in 1995 as *The Fundamental Concepts of Metaphysics: World, Finitude, Solitude*, Heidegger moved away from a focus on the centrality of anxiety and instead presented boredom as a *Grundstimmung*, or 'fundamental attunement'.[5] Most importantly this attunement of boredom was presented by Heidegger, in this lecture series, as historically *situated*. Thus, even in the late 1920s, Heidegger was moving towards the idea that different periods of history have been associated with different moods, what he called 'epochal attunements'. However, a number of commentators make a case that in the course of his writing on technology and nihilism (see below) anxiety again emerges, this time not as a universal state-of-mind of every individual Dasein, but as the characteristic mood of modernity. For example, Dreyfus writes that:

> Later Heidegger . . . gives up his existential account of anxiety, and of falling as a motivated cover-up of Dasein's essential nullity and unsettledness . . . Heidegger the thinker (not the hermeneutic phenomenologist with a preontological understanding of the sense of being) interprets anxiety as a specific response to the rootlessness of the contemporary technological world.
>
> (Dreyfus 1991: 336–37)

However, there is little textual elaboration of this connection between anxiety and modernity in the later works of Heidegger himself.[6] Michel Haar (1992) makes the point that Heidegger speaks more about a mood of 'terror' in relation to the nihilism of modernity, but whether this can be directly equated with anxiety remains unclear. I will not dwell on the issue here. My purpose in introducing Heidegger's concept of 'epochal attunements' is meant merely to support my use of the insights of *Being and Time*, minus the concept of existential anxiety as a universal. My argument is that the connection between anxiety, death and authenticity presented in *Being and Time* as a fundamental aspect of human life is, in fact, something which is particularly associated with modernity and thus not universal. In the next chapter I will turn to the work of sociologists and philosophers other than Heidegger to make my case for a specific connection between anxiety and modernity. However, in the rest of this chapter I will use Heidegger's critique of modernity as a way into this issue. This critique is also relevant to the themes of Chapter 10 and the question of how we should respond to anxiety.

The later works of Heidegger

While Heidegger makes it clear at the beginning of *Being and Time* that his exploration of Dasein is only a path into the exploration of being itself, this path was the only one opened in the work. In his writings after the mid-1930s, Heidegger spoke less about exploring being through an exploration of Dasein and more about exploring being in a more direct way. In this vision human existence and temporality arise within a wider, more encompassing, 'openness' which cannot be grasped in terms of human reality alone. Heidegger began to attempt a 'thinking' of being in its own terms. As Zimmerman remarks, this was a move away from the 'remaining anthropocentrism' (Zimmerman 1993) discernible in the earlier works. The later works increasingly focused on language as having a direct relationship to being outside the confines of ordinary human life. Heidegger also increasingly turned his attention to the history of being. In the rest of this chapter I shall focus on these writings, and on his reflections about technology developed in the 1950s.

In a series of deconstructive readings of the great thinkers of the Western metaphysical tradition he sought to disclose the underlying and unthought presuppositions of this tradition. For Heidegger, the history of metaphysics was about the way in which the question of being had been 'forgotten'. In the 1949 essay 'The way back into the ground of metaphysics' he draws on a metaphor from Descartes in which the whole of philosophy is likened to a tree. In this metaphor, the roots are metaphysics and the trunk is physics, while the other disciplines emerge from these central structures as do the branches of a tree. Heidegger seizes upon this image and asks:

> In what soil do the roots of the tree of philosophy have their hold? Out of what ground do the roots – and through them the whole tree – receive their nourishing juices and strengths?

In other words:

> What is the basis and element of metaphysics? What is metaphysics,
> viewed from its ground? What is metaphysics itself, at bottom?
>
> (Heidegger 1956: 207)

His point is that philosophy systematically forgets the ground, even
though the ground always enters and lives in the roots themselves and
indeed in the tree as a whole. Whenever metaphysics thinks about beings
as beings, then such beings are 'already in sight'. What shows them up as
beings in the first place is ignored by philosophy. Heidegger's complaint is
that metaphysics, far from revealing the ground from which our thinking
has sprung, actually works to conceal this ground:

> Due to the manner in which it thinks of beings, metaphysics almost
> seems to be, without knowing it, the barrier which keeps man from the
> original involvement of Being in human nature.
>
> (Heidegger 1956: 211)

Heidegger's historical works attempt to show how the ground, i.e.
being itself, has been 'revealed' in its 'concealment' by metaphysics. He
moves away from a vision of Dasein as some sort of fixed opening to
being. Instead, he historicizes the notion of Dasein's clearing. Thus,
Dasein is seen to be historically the recipient of a succession of different
clearings.

My presentation of Heidegger's later philosophy will not attempt, in
any way, to be comprehensive. However, as these ideas have substantially
influenced the other philosophers whose works are discussed in the next
section, it is important to provide at least an introduction to this
philosophy. I am also concerned to show how the role of anxiety changed
in his thought. In addition, in Chapter 10 I shall make use of the concept
of *Gelassenheit* (releasement) that emerges from his writing on
technology.

Heidegger's history of being and the critique of modernity

In his 1938 essay 'The age of the world picture' Heidegger asks the
question, 'What is the essence of the modern age?' He answers that
modern times can be characterized as the era of the 'world picture'
(*Weltbild*). He uses the word 'picture' as it is used in the expression, 'We
get the picture.' This phrase indicates that whatever is, or whatever is

happening, is somehow set out before us and we are equipped and prepared for it. Heidegger says:

> Where the world becomes picture, what is, in its entirety, is juxtaposed
> as that for which man is prepared and which, correspondingly, he
> therefore intends to bring before himself and have before himself, and
> consequently intends in a decisive sense to set in place before himself.
>
> (Heidegger 1977: 129)

In the modern era, the Age of the World Picture, everything that is, including ourselves, shows up for us as resources to be utilized, enhanced, transformed or ordered for the sake of greater and greater efficiency. In contrast, in the medieval era the world was not experienced in the form of a picture standing before us and to which we had ready access. Instead, in the Middle Ages:

> . . . that which is, is the *ens creatum*, that which is created by the
> personal Creator-God as the highest cause. Here, to be in being means
> to belong within a specific rank of the order of what has been created.
>
> (Heidegger 1977: 130)

For medieval Christians, reality was the presence of created entities – beings which were 'finished products' (Dreyfus 1991: 338). Human beings stood in a position of acceptance with regard to the world, and knowledge was about understanding the order of creation. Heidegger also contrasts the modern age with that of the ancient Greeks. For the Greeks, the world was not there as a 'picture' for human beings to order for their purposes. In contrast, it was the world, being itself, that looked upon human beings and which opened itself to them. Humanity was:

> . . . gathered towards presencing, by that which opens itself. To be
> beheld by what is, to be included and maintained within its openness
> and in that way to be borne along by it, to be driven about by its opposi-
> tions and marked by its discord – that is the essence of man in the great
> age of the Greeks.
>
> (Heidegger 1977: 131)

In these different ages there were different understandings of being and thus different conceptions of metaphysics. In spite of the fact that Heidegger finds echoes of the modern approach to reality in works of Protagoras, Plato and Aristotle, he argues that they all remain within the general framework of the 'Greek fundamental experience of what is'. It is only because their thought has been presented to us through a 'modern humanistic interpretation'- that we have failed to realize how different their approach to being really is. He says it has been denied to us to:

> ... ponder the Being that opened itself to Greek antiquity in such a way as to leave to it its uniqueness and strangeness.
>
> (Heidegger 1977: 144)

For modern humanity the possibility of experiencing being in this way has disappeared. Because our understanding of being is that of the world picture, beings show up for us simply as objects to be controlled and organized according to our agendas. Ours is the age of technology.

Technology and nihilism

In his essay 'The question concerning technology', Heidegger argues that to grasp the importance of modern technology fully it is not enough to understand it merely as a 'means' to an end: rather, we need an ontological understanding in which technology becomes a mode of 'revealing' being. He traces the origins of the word 'technology' to the Greek *technikon*, which in turn means that which belongs to *techne*. This term refers on the one hand to the activities and skills of the craftsman, and on the other, to 'the arts of the mind and the fine arts'. Furthermore:

> From the earliest times until Plato the word *techne* is linked with the word *episteme*. Both words are names for knowing in the widest sense. They mean to be entirely at home in something, to understand and be expert in it. Such knowing provides an opening up. As an opening up it is a revealing.
>
> (Heidegger 1977: 13)

Technology is the modern cultural paradigm. It is the context in which the world as 'world picture' comes into view. This understanding of the concept of technology is extremely important because, as Dreyfus points out, Heidegger is sometimes presented as a latter day Luddite who simply wishes to turn the clock back (Dreyfus 1993: 304). Heidegger does not ask the question, 'How can we control technology?' In fact, responding to modern technology in this way is part of the problem. It is a response set by the nature of technology itself. Understanding our predicament as something to be solved by more appropriate *controls* is itself a technological response:

> The instrumental conception of technology conditions every attempt to bring man into the right relation to technology . . . The will to mastery becomes all the more urgent the more technology threatens to slip from human control.
>
> (Heidegger 1977: 5)

Heidegger's concern is not with the destructive effects of specific technologies but with the larger human implications of living in an age whose metaphysics is brought into being by technology. In 'The question concerning technology', echoing his earlier reflections on the concept of the 'world picture', Heidegger also introduces the term *Gestell*. Lovitt translates this as 'Enframing' and adds in a footnote that he uses the prefix 'en-' to give a sense of the active meaning Heidegger gives to the German word. Lovitt says:

> . . . the reader should be careful not to interpret the word as though it simply meant a framework of some sort. Instead he should constantly remember that Enframing is fundamentally a calling forth. It is a 'challenging claim', a demanding summons, that 'gathers' so as to reveal. This claim *enframes* in that it assembles and orders. It puts into a framework or configuration everything that it summons forth, through an ordering for use that it is forever restructuring anew.
>
> (Lovitt, footnote in Heidegger 1977: 19)

Heidegger introduces the word *Gestell* 'as the name for the essence of modern technology'. Thus Heidegger uses the term with a specific sense: it refers to the sort of ordering of the world *for human purposes* that is characteristic of the modern era. Previous epochs of Western history were not characterized by this type of Enframing. He argues that Enframing as a way of human beings relating to their world actually predates the rise of technology itself. Thus Enframing is not the result of actual technologies, rather it would appear that the former gives rise to the latter. Enframing involves both 'attitude and behaviour' and can be seen first in European society in the rise of the scientific approach to nature:

> Accordingly, man's ordering attitude and behaviour display themselves first in the rise of modern physics as an exact science. Modern science's way of representing pursues and entraps nature as a calculable coherence of forces. Modern physics is not experimental physics because it applies apparatus to the questioning of nature. Rather the reverse is true. Because physics, indeed already as pure theory sets nature up to exhibit itself as a coherence of forces calculable in advance, it therefore orders its experiments precisely for the purpose of asking whether and how nature reports itself when set up in this way.
>
> (Heidegger 1977: 21)

In other words, modern physics does not simply encounter the natural world and then develop ways of investigating it. The notion that it would be appropriate to 'investigate' nature happens first and on the basis of this particular understanding of the natural world it then becomes possible to think in terms of scientific investigation. Enframing involves, in a profound way, the domination of a certain type of thought. In this, Dasein comes to have a particular relationship with the entities of the world in which they become resources for it. These entities include fellow human beings. Olafson writes:

> Technological thought treats everything as being an object of one kind or another, and it does so because it is in this form that the world corresponds to the disposition to manipulate and control it. This disposition is observable in spheres of life as apparently remote from one another as philosophy and the technologies of management. What is common to these very different domains is a growing determination to decide in terms of a pragmatic a priori what kinds of entities are to be recognized as existing for the purposes of a given activity.
>
> (Olafson 1987: 215–16)

Heidegger warns about this ever-increasing expansion of calculative and objectifying thought in the *Discourse on Thinking* and suggests that the 'greatest danger' facing humanity in the modern epoch is that:

> . . . the approaching tide of technological revolution in the atomic age could so captivate, bewitch, dazzle, and beguile man that calculative thinking may someday come to be accepted and practised *as the only way* of thinking.
>
> (Heidegger 1966: 56)

What is at stake is not a problem to be solved but an ontological question concerning our modern understanding of being.

In the essay 'The word of Nietzsche: "God is dead"', Heidegger, following on from Nietzsche and Kierkegaard, further characterizes the modern era as the age of nihilism. In the modern age, the technological age, the era of the 'world picture', being is experienced as nothing but a manifestation of the will to power. Being is thus denied its dimensionality. Unlike Nietzsche, however, Heidegger does not regard the 'death of God' as the cause of nihilism, but sees it rather the other way around. Nihilism is the 'world-historical movement of the peoples of the earth who have been drawn into the power realm of the modern age' (Heidegger 1977: 63) and is, in its essence, the negation of being. For Heidegger, when human beings understand the world as being composed of resources that can be used in more or less interchangeable ways, choices and decisions emerge about alternative ways of using these resources. These choices depend on what we wish to use the resources for. This can only be determined by further calculative reasoning. To do this, we have to articulate what is at issue for us in any given situation. In this process, we generate the 'values' that will guide our calculations and decisions. As Joseph Rouse writes:

> This is the significance of the concept of 'value': it transforms the config-
> uration of practices within which thought and action are intelligible to
> us into something we can reckon with and wilfully implement. When
> this happens, however, the values chosen do not govern our choice, for
> they are what is chosen. That for the sake of which our choice of values
> is made always withdraws from calculative awareness. This complication
> calls for further reckoning, in a futile attempt to disclose our 'ultimate'
> values.
>   (Rouse 1987: 261)

For Heidegger, this leads to an endless expansion of calculative thought. What is at stake is a will towards mastery and control, not just of the world around us, but also of ourselves. This is similar to Nietzsche's 'will to power'. We have entered an era of nihilism and within modernity there is no longer any stable structure to what is at stake for us. Power, as expressed in the calculative thought of our times, robs us of any coherent and generally accepted meaning for our lives. In a section that will be echoed later by Foucault, Heidegger writes in *Nietzsche, Volume IV: Nihilism*:

> The new valuation . . . supplants all earlier values with power, the
> uppermost value, but first and foremost because power and *only power*
> posits values, validates them, and makes decisions about the possible
> justifications of a valuation . . . To the extent that it is truly power, alone
> determining all beings, power does not recognize the worth or value of
> anything outside of itself.
>   (Heidegger 1982: 7)

Subjectivity and modernity

Heidegger argues that Descartes stands at the beginning of the modern era in metaphysics. In his metaphysics the self becomes an 'ego-logical self' and enters a relationship of representation with that which it has positioned before itself. Thus the strong sense of objectivity brought into being in the modern era is linked to a strong sense of the subjective. Olafson contrasts the later Heidegger's engagement with Descartes with the arguments developed in *Being and Time*. In the earlier work Heidegger criticized Descartes' separation of the inner mind from an exterior world. He argued that this actually passed over how the world is really experienced by Dasein. As we have seen in Chapter 5, Heidegger was of the opinion that Descartes' move in this was a major source of diffi-culties for subsequent Western philosophy. When Heidegger returned to

Descartes, in the context of his writing about Nietzsche, he was more concerned by the latter's positioning of the self as the pre-eminent entity:

> Heidegger emphasizes instead what he takes to be the characteristic effort of modern thought to elevate the thinking self to the status of the preeminent and ultimately exclusive self for which all other entities that in medieval parlance were 'subjects' on an equal footing with it become 'objects'.
>
> (Olafson 1987: 212)

The era of the 'world picture' is also the era of the glorified self. It is the age of humanism. For Heidegger, humanism:

> . . . designates that philosophical interpretation of man which explains and evaluates whatever is, in its entirety, from the standpoint of man and in relation to man.
>
> (Heidegger 1977: 133)

This has brought into being a self that can best be described as 'pathologically hypertrophied'.[7] Its exaltation as the source of everything also renders it fragile and precarious. In a situation where human being has become the sole source of meaning and order in the world and at the same time has become increasingly self-conscious and separate from the world, there is a continuous tendency for humanity to feel disconnected and for the meaning of the world to appear arbitrary and unconvincing. Heidegger speaks about the 'oblivion of Being' and in the 1949 essay referred to above, 'The way back into the ground of metaphysics', appears to make a specific connection between this 'oblivion' and the state of anxiety (anxiety is here translated as 'dread'):

> If the oblivion of Being which has been described here should be real, would there not be occasion enough for a thinker who recalls Being to experience a genuine horror? What more can his thinking do than to endure in dread this fateful withdrawal while first of all facing up to the oblivion of Being?
>
> (Heidegger 1956: 211–12)

Furthermore, this oblivion is ever-increasing. As our involvement with technology increases and ever more aspects of our lives are structured and ordered according to an ethic of efficiency our thinking becomes almost exclusively calculative. Heidegger asks:

> What if the absence of this involvement (of Being in human nature) and the oblivion of this absence determined the entire modern age? What if the absence of Being abandoned man more and more exclusively to

beings, leaving him forsaken and far from any involvement of Being in
his nature, while this forsakenness itself remained veiled? What if this
were the case – and had been the case for a long time now? What if there
were signs that this oblivion will become still more decisive in the
future?

(Heidegger 1977: 211)

Summary

In the later philosophy, Heidegger moved away from an attempt to
provide a 'fundamental ontology', a universal description of the make-up
of human reality. Instead, he presents the characteristics of Dasein
described in *Being and Time* as possible attributes of a human being –
they are no longer necessary features of our make-up. Human reality is
understood as having different attunements in different epochs and
having different relationships with being in these different epochs. As
Richard Polt notes, Heidegger's style of writing and the language he uses
also change (Polt 1999: 119). There is a move away from the technical,
almost scientific vocabulary of *Being and Time* towards a more poetic and
sometimes mystical set of words and phrases.

The later writings also signal a shift in Heidegger's approach to the
question of anxiety. This changes from being a fundamental mood that
confronts Dasein with a sense of nothingness and thus opens up the possibility of an authentic mode of living. As we have seen above, the mood
anxiety does not feature to any great extent in the later works. However,
Heidegger's writings about technology and modernity continue to focus
on a sense of human homelessness and alienation in the world. In the
'Letter on humanism' Heidegger praises Marx for his identification of 'the
estrangement of man' (Heidegger 1993: 243). On this account, although
Heidegger decries any 'naive notions of materialism' and wants to derive
this sense of estrangement from a deeper metaphysical homelessness, he
says that Marx's view of history is superior to others. I shall mention
Marx's understanding of alienation again in the next chapter. This will be
part of a discussion of the social dynamics of modernity and
postmodernity.

Meaning and the culture of postmodernity

Chapter 9
Modernity, postmodernity and the question of meaning

Introduction

I will now discuss the work of other writers (philosophers and social theorists) who have written on the subjects of alienation, anxiety and meaninglessness. In this section, I am moving from philosophy towards sociology. I shall begin with a discussion of some ideas from the philosophers Charles Taylor and Paul Tillich. I shall then mention Marx's concept of alienation and this shall lead to the work of the sociologist Anthony Giddens and others. The questions I am asking in this chapter are as follows. Are there aspects of our contemporary Western cultures which mean that we have a particular vulnerability with regard to anxiety and meaninglessness? Has the move to postmodernity made this more extreme? Could the current preoccupation with trauma stem from this vulnerability? In the next chapter I shall ask how can we best respond to post-traumatic anxiety in the light of this analysis.

As should be clear by now, I do not believe that these questions can be answered simply by referring to an epidemiological literature. This is predicated upon the assumptions of Western psychology and psychiatry as outlined in Chapter 2. This literature assumes the universal validity of modern Western diagnostic categories and fits the various worlds it encounters into these. The problem being raised by this book is that this 'fitting' is, in fact, a forced fitting. The leading cross-cultural psychiatrist Arthur Kleinman argues that psychiatry's concern to construct reliable diagnostic 'instruments' for use in different cultural groups simply misses the point. He says that the use of such instruments in different situations cannot by itself lead to any valid conclusions about the nature of psychiatric disorders in such different settings. The possibility of making a *category fallacy* is inherent in such an approach. According to Kleinman:

> A category fallacy is the reification of a nosological category developed
> for a particular cultural group that is then applied to members of

another culture for whom it lacks coherence and its validity has not been established.

(Kleinman 1987: 452)

When it comes to the literature on trauma, what is at stake is the massive rise in interest, both clinically and culturally, in the phenomenon in the past 20 years. We have seen in Chapter 4 how Judith Herman argues that trauma and its effects have only become visible in Western societies in recent years because of the rise of the feminist movement and campaigns against the war in Vietnam. Her position is that PTSD, as understood by modern psychiatry, has always existed but has been pushed out of view until recently on account of the patriarchal nature of society. If this was the case, then there might be some mileage in using diagnostic instruments (centred on the concept of PTSD) cross-culturally. In Herman's account, echoed by most trauma researchers, PTSD has universal validity. However, in Chapter 4 we also examined the work of the anthropologist Allan Young who presents a very different account of the emergence of PTSD. I believe that Young's arguments are persuasive, and by now I hope to have added to his position by showing that there *are* important philosophical assumptions underlying the discourse on trauma. If the reader accepts this then he/she will acknowledge that there will be problems with the use of the PTSD framework cross-culturally and trans-historically.

This means that we cannot answer the question about the relationship, if any, between trauma and modernity/postmodernity through scientific analysis alone. The massive rise of interest in trauma in Western societies is a fact. The massive rise in patients diagnosed as suffering from PTSD is a fact. If my analysis in Section II was correct and there is an ontological dimension to the phenomenon of post-traumatic anxiety then these facts will not be fully explained through science alone. This question cries out for an exploration that is not premised on the positivist assumptions discussed in Chapter 1. What I present in this chapter is a discussion of philosophical and sociological writing which I believe supports a linkage between the move to postmodernity and the rise of post-traumatic anxiety and the associated medical discourse around trauma. My intention is not to prove this linkage but to move the debate about trauma and its sequelae away from a narrow 'medical' and individualistic focus on PTSD and towards an understanding of trauma as a social and cultural phenomenon through and through.

Modernity and the question of meaning

I have already discussed the work of the philosopher Charles Taylor in Chapter 5. In other writing, Taylor draws attention to the ways in which modern perspectives in areas of ethical concern have been in a position of mutual support to Enlightenment ideas about the importance and centrality of reason in human affairs. In his book *Sources of the Self: The Making of the Modern Identity* (1989), Taylor aims to articulate some of the background assumptions implicit in our moral beliefs. He is engaged in what he calls a 'moral ontology'. Whilst I am wary of the universalism inherent in Taylor's position I think his framework is a useful starting point for some comparative work. He argues that in every culture there are basically three axes along which one can examine assumptions about morality. However, there are great differences in how these axes and issues are conceived, how they relate to one another and their relative importance to different cultures. These axes are:

1. respect for human life
2. what constitutes a good and meaningful life
3. the notion of personal dignity.

The first of these concerns the moral beliefs around our sense that human life is to be respected. Every culture has a different notion of what this involves and there are different prohibitions and obligations in this respect. For some cultures the definition of who is part of the 'human race' may not correspond with current Western universalism, but nevertheless it would appear that every society has rules that involve prohibitions against killing and harming fellow 'humans'. In the Western world the issues surrounding this particular moral axis have recently been formulated in terms of rights. The second concerns the issue of what kind of life is worth living, of what constitutes a rich, meaningful life as opposed to one concerned with merely secondary matters or trivia. The third issue of dignity refers to our sense of ourselves as commanding attitudinal respect from others.

Taylor argues that this third axis was the most important in the morality of ancient Greece. He suggests that for us this is difficult to conceive as it seems obvious that the first axis is paramount, followed by the second. However, what is important to our discussion here is his observation that:

> . . . one of the most important ways in which our age stands out from earlier ones concerns the second axis. A set of questions makes sense to us which turn around the meaning of life and which would not have been fully understandable in earlier epochs. Moderns can anxiously doubt whether life has meaning, or wonder what its meaning is. However philosophers may be inclined to attack these formulations as vague or confused, the fact remains that we all have an immediate sense of what kind of worry is being articulated in these words.
>
> (Taylor 1989: 16)

While questions along the second axis can arise for different people in different cultures, for people living in modern society they have a particular depth and a particular set of implications. Taylor points out that someone living in a warrior society might well ask whether his tale of courageous deeds lives up to the promise of his lineage or the demands of his station in life. On the other hand, people living in a very strongly religious community will often ask whether the demand for piety means that they should change their life or follow a call to some purer more dedicated vocation. The point is, however, that in each of these scenarios some framework stands in the background unquestioned. This framework helps define the demands by which such people measure their lives with regards to its fullness or its emptiness. For us, however, living in the contemporary Western world, there are no such shared frameworks that might serve as a background for the articulation of such questions. Taylor says:

> . . . the problem of the meaning of life is therefore on our agenda, however much we may jibe at this phrase, either in the form of a threatened loss of meaning or because making sense of our life is the object of a quest. And those whose spiritual agenda is mainly defined in this way are in a fundamentally different existential predicament from that which dominated most previous cultures and still defines the lives of people today.
>
> (Taylor 1989: 18)

Taylor then makes a point that is very relevant to our discussion about anxiety. He points out that the anxiety that is experienced in a strongly religious community where the unchallenged framework makes demands that we fear being unable to meet is something very different from an anxiety associated with a sense of meaninglessness. He points to the anguish experienced by Luther with regard to questions of faith. Luther's struggle, and his sense of inescapable condemnation, were quite clearly profoundly painful. But however one might want to describe Luther's crisis it was not a crisis of meaning. Taylor makes the point that:

> . . . the existential predicament in which one fears condemnation is quite different from the one where one fears, above all, meaninglessness. The dominance of the latter perhaps defines our age.
>
> In a way which we cannot yet properly understand, the shift between these two existential predicaments seems to be matched by a recent change in the dominant patterns of psychopathology.
>
> (Taylor 1989: 18–19)

Taylor's arguments about the moral ontology of the modern self are, I believe, quite close to those developed by Heidegger and are overtly in support of the connections I am making here. I am particularly intrigued by this last comment about the 'dominant patterns of psychopathology'. I shall return to this issue at the end of this chapter.

The descriptions of anxiety in Paul Tillich's book *The Courage to Be* (1952) are also consonant with what I am suggesting and his historical framework is shared with both Heidegger and Taylor. Writing about courage, which he says is usually described as the power of the mind to overcome fear, Tillich says that in the twentieth century fear itself has undergone close scrutiny. In particular, he notes the distinction, made by Heidegger and others (and discussed in Chapter 7), between fear and anxiety. Fear is held to be in relation to something tangible in the world, whereas anxiety is in relation to a threat to the coherence of the world as a whole. Tillich suggests that anxiety tends to hide itself in fear, as in fear the tangible object can at least be faced by courage. As our time has become known as the 'age of anxiety', according to Tillich, courage has become the ability to overcome anxiety. With this in mind, Tillich develops what he terms an 'ontology of anxiety'. Echoing Heidegger, he defines anxiety as 'the state in which a being is aware of its possible nonbeing'. He also says: 'anxiety is the existential awareness of nonbeing' (Tillich 1952: 35). Tillich's approach to the existential dimension of anxiety is quite close to that of Heidegger in *Being and Time*. Thus, for Tillich, anxiety is an inevitable part of being a human being. Anxiety is an existential universal; it belongs to existence as such, and not to any particular pathological state of mind. Likewise, and unlike the later Heidegger, anxiety occurs trans-historically and in different cultures. However, according to Tillich's analysis, because anxiety is, in effect, the threat of nonbeing, and nonbeing has different qualities, it is possible to think of existential anxiety as having different dimensions. He argues that there are three 'directions' from which nonbeing threatens being. The first of these involves threats to man's 'ontic self-affirmation'. These can be of a relative nature, involving issues of fate, or of an absolute nature, in the form of death. Second, nonbeing can threaten man's 'spiritual self-affirmation' which again can be relative, in terms of emptiness, or absolute, in terms of meaninglessness. Lastly, nonbeing can pose a threat to man's 'moral self-affirmation'. Relatively, this can take the form of guilt, and absolutely it can appear as condemnation. Corresponding to this threefold threat, anxiety can appear as:

> ... that of fate and death (briefly, the anxiety of death), that of emptiness and loss of meaning (briefly, the anxiety of meaninglessness), that of guilt and condemnation (briefly, the anxiety of condemnation).
> (Tillich 1952: 41)

According to Tillich, while these three forms of existential anxiety are not mutually exclusive and can appear together, in different historical epochs it is usual for one form to be dominant. The anxiety of fate and death is the most universal and the most basic. Human beings are always, and every-where, anxiously aware of the threat of nonbeing and need courage to endure. While this threat is absolute in the threat of death and only relative in the threat of fate, in reality fate can only threaten us because death is in the background. Again, echoing Heidegger, Tillich writes that the threat of death pervades our lives as human beings. It is what gives power and impact to the other fateful contingencies of our lives. This form of anxiety dominated Western civilization in the 'ancient' period. Tillich provides an account of this in relation to the courage displayed by the Stoics and notes that although the anxiety of fate and death was dominant in this period, the other forms of anxiety were also present. At the end of the Middle Ages, anxiety of guilt and condemnation became most prominent. The threat of condemnation is very visible in the works of art of the pre-Reformation and Reformation periods. Images of hell and purgatory abound. Christian Europe witnessed a proliferation of various ways of alleviating this anxiety. Pilgrimages to holy places, devotion to shrines and relics, rituals of confession and penitence all became very common. In this time, the anxiety surrounding death was joined by an extreme concern about sin and its effects. Tillich remarks that 'death and the devil were allied in the anxious imagination of the period' (1952: 59). While questions of spiritual doubt did emerge at times, in particular during the course of the Renaissance and the Reformation, the anxiety of condemnation remained dominant throughout this epoch and it is only with the Enlightenment and the rise of humanism that concern about spiritual nonbeing became prominent. Tillich writes:

> . . . the breakdown of absolutism, the development of Liberalism and Democracy, the rise of a technical civilization . . . its victory over all enemies and its own beginning disintegration – these are the socio-logical presuppositions for the third main period of anxiety. In this the anxiety of emptiness and meaninglessness is dominant. We are under the threat of spiritual non being.
>
> (Tillich 1952: 61–62)

Concern about emptiness and meaninglessness are the central anxieties of our time. As noted above, Tillich relates these forms of anxiety directly to questions of 'spiritual self-affirmation'. Meaninglessness is the absolute threat of nonbeing to human spirituality, and emptiness is the relative version of this. The former is anxiety about the 'loss of an ultimate concern', the loss of a 'spiritual centre' that gives an ultimate sense of coherence, order and purpose to the world. In this, there is the loss of any answer to the question of life's meaning. The anxiety of emptiness

> . . . is aroused by the threat of nonbeing to the special contents of the spiritual life. A belief breaks down through external events or inner processes: one is cut off from creative participation in a sphere of culture, one feels frustrated about something which one had passionately affirmed, one is driven from devotion to one object to devotion to another and again on to another, because the meaning of each of them vanishes and the creative eros is transformed into indifference or aversion.
>
> (Tillich 1952: 47–48)

However, a 'spiritual centre' cannot simply be created. It cannot be produced 'intentionally'. Indeed, attempts to do so produce deeper anxiety: 'the anxiety of emptiness drives us to the abyss of meaninglessness' (1952: 48).

Thus, Heidegger's discussion of how anxiety, characterized by dislocation and loss of meaning, is particularly associated with modern times is supported by a number of other philosophers. The psychotherapist Rollo May, who in his book *The Meaning of Anxiety* (1977) was substantially influenced by the work of Tillich, also talks about the loss of a meaningful world and the connection of this with the problem of anxiety. We shall examine May's existentialist response to this predicament in the next chapter when we contrast this response to that of Heidegger and other philosophers. May argues that:

> [the] quantity of anxiety prevalent in the present period arises from the fact that the values and standards underlying modern culture are themselves threatened . . . The threats involved in the present social changes are not threats which can be met on the basis of the assumptions of the culture but rather are threats to those underlying assumptions themselves.
>
> (May 1977: 238)

Marx and the question of alienation

Moving to a somewhat different perspective, we saw at the end of the last chapter how Heidegger made a connection between his own sense of metaphysical homelessness and Marx's writing on alienation. This is a theme present throughout Marx's work and is a central plank of his critique of capitalism. However, it is discussed at most length in the *Economic and Social Manuscripts* of 1844. In this work, Marx argues that capitalism fundamentally involves a process of exploitation where the product of a worker's labour is not only taken from him but set to work against him by increasing the power of the employer. He criticizes the political economists of his day who present concepts such as the 'market', 'commodities', 'exchange value' and 'capital' as though they were simply objective aspects of the economy, having a life independent of human mediation. This presentation conceals the fact that these phenomena are actually the products of real human and social relationships. Marx wants to show that all economic phenomena are actually socially produced. The 'market' is a human construct with human benefits and human costs. Economists systematically obscure this fact and in so doing conceal the class nature of capitalist societies.

Under conditions of capitalism, the worker is alienated from the product of his work and from his own productive activity. He finds that what he has made is not his. It becomes instead an 'objectification', 'a power independent of the producer'. The worker relates to the product of his work as to an alien object. The worker does not own and is no longer involved with the object he produces. This is obviously different to the situation of an artist or of a worker within the craft guilds of the pre-capitalist period. Marx says that the worker in capitalist society 'puts his life into the object' and as this is not his so too his life is not his:

> So the greater this product the less he is himself. The externalization of the worker in his product implies not only that his labour becomes an object, an exterior existence but that it also exists outside him, independent and alien, and becomes a self-sufficient power opposite him, that the life that he has lent to the object affronts him, hostile and alien.
>
> (Marx, in McLellan 1977: 79)

But, he says, alienation shows itself not simply in the object but also in the work of production itself. In capitalist economies work does not belong to the worker. Because the object of his labour is alien to him, his labour itself becomes alien to him. He makes the point that work is obviously alien to the worker because when there is no 'physical or other compulsion, labour is avoided like the plague' (Marx, in McLellan 1977: 80). These aspects of alienation lead to others, and in the end man becomes alienated from man. As social beings, our relationships, our beliefs, our pains and our pleasures are all bound up with the sort of economy and society in which we live. Under capitalism, based as it is on the alienation of the worker from both the object of his work and from his labour itself, we become an alienated 'species'. Human relationships become reduced to the operations of the market. Our lives and our values become bound up with the importance of money, as this is what is received in lieu of labour.

From the point of our discussion about alienation and subjectivity in the modern period, of greatest importance is Marx's derivation of the reality of private property and with it the separation of the individual from the social, *from* the alienation of capitalist forms of production. This is directly contrary to the prevailing analysis of the political economists who put the development of private property as the origin of capitalist production. For Marx, private property is the result of the alienation involved in production. He says:

> Through alienated labour, then, man creates not only his relationship to the object and act of production as to alien and hostile men; he creates too the relationship in which other men stand to his production and his product and the relationship in which he stands to these other men. Just as he turns his production into his own loss of reality and punishment and his own product into a loss, a product that does not belong to him, so he creates the domination of the man who does not produce over the production and the product. As he alienates his activity from himself, so he hands over to an alien person an activity that does not belong to him.
>
> (Marx, in McLellan 1977: 84)

For Marx, private property is the result of 'externalized labour'. Capitalist forms of production give rise to alienated labour that, in turn, gives rise to private property. With these arise a discourse of needs and rights centred on the individual as something separate from the society in which he/she is located. Traditional political economy begins with the isolated individual self and ignores the social relations that stand behind this idea.

Thus, for Marx our modern sense of estrangement arises very clearly from the conditions of production and the fact that the product of the worker's labour is something that becomes external and alien to him/her. As we shall see below, a number of sociologists view the move from modernity to postmodernity as the result of a change in the focus of capitalism from production to consumption. The suggestion is that this move has led to further forms of alienation.

The move to postmodernity

I wish now to discuss cultural aspects of the move from modernity to postmodernity.[1] I am aware that the latter term is contended in its references and somewhat nebulous in its actual usage. However, it has been used now for many years and appears to be here to stay. However, at this point it is important to restate the distinction made in Chapter 1 between, on the one hand, the term 'postmodernity' as used to refer to a contemporary social, cultural and political *condition*, something we simply find ourselves in the midst of, and, on the other hand, the use of the term 'postmodern', in a more positive way, to refer to a *way of reflecting* upon the world and our place within it.

In the next chapter I shall explore this second meaning of the term. Here, I wish to focus on the postmodern condition as a cultural epoch, as a way of life. I will suggest that, in this way of life, whatever systems of order and coherence came in the wake of modernity have now begun to disappear.

Just as the past two decades have witnessed an enormous growth in the literature pertaining to trauma and PTSD, so too in the same period we have seen 'postmodernity' emerge as a central preoccupation of cultural studies and the various branches of social theory.[2] In the last chapter I discussed some of the major cultural developments within modernity. These were the move to an ontology that was characterized by Heidegger as involving 'the oblivion of being'. The second, and intimately related, development was the emergence of what I called 'pathologically hypertrophied subjectivity'. In Heidegger's analysis, both of these developments have given rise to the nihilism of modernity. In turn, this nihilism has been related to the mood of anxiety by a number of philosophers and sociologists. This (Heideggerian) anxiety, which I said resonated with descriptions of post-traumatic anxiety in Chapter 7, is thus something particularly associated with the culture of modernity. By showing how these developments have become even more acute within postmodernity I hope to develop a convincing, if not scientific, account of how post-traumatic anxiety has become a preoccupation of our times. I will examine the implications of this account in the next chapter and in the conclusion.

The decline of 'meaning' within postmodernity

One of the central goals of what I termed the 'Enlightenment project' in Chapter 2 was to use reason in the pursuit of an efficient and orderly society. Modernity was to incorporate a social life established according to the dictates of science and rational planning. An orderly society was to be a goal in itself. In the utilitarian calculations of modern times the best society would be one that was predictable and orderly. However, as Zygmunt Bauman writes:

> Among the multitude of impossible tasks that modernity set itself and that made modernity into what it is, the task of order (more precisely and most importantly, of *order as a task*) stands out – as the least possible among the impossible and the least disposable among the indispensable; indeed, as the archetype for all other tasks, one that renders all other tasks mere metaphors of itself.
>
> (Bauman 1991: 4)

Thus, even within modernity order was an impossible dream. Disorder always seems to follow in its wake. Indeed, order and disorder appear as twin concepts and the idea of an orderly society, free from chaos and conflict, was, surely, one of the greatest illusions of modernity. As we pass into the state of postmodernity, disorder becomes integral to our very ways of life. Indeed, in the postmodern cultural arena 'meaning' itself is systematically undermined. In writing 'a political economy of postmodernism', Scott Lash talks about 'the decline of meaning' in economic terms:

> Meaning is only achieved by the connection of signifieds to signifiers. If there is an oversupply of such signifiers – as there appears to be in today's constant bombardment of images and sounds – and only a finite number of signifieds to go round, then large numbers of signifiers will persist with no meanings attached, and be literally experienced as such.

> (Lash 1990: 43)

Within postmodernity, we experience reality as fleeting and unstable. The meaningful connections of our social world are rendered fragile. Elements of the everyday culture itself seem to work to destroy predictability and meaning. This is a theme Anthony Giddens returns to in a number of works. In his book *Modernity and Self-Identity: Self and Society in the Late Modern Age* (1991), he writes specifically about the position of the self in a 'runaway world'. One of the key features of modernity that makes it different from what Giddens refers to as 'traditional society', is its extreme dynamism. Not only is the *pace* of social change more rapid than at any other time but the *scope* of this change and its *profound* nature mean that modernity contrasts markedly with other cultural systems. Giddens describes three elements involved in this dynamism. The first of these involves the separation of time and space. In the global world of post- or late-modernity telecommunications technology means that time is increasingly set apart from geography. Media events, such as rock concerts and sporting events, are experienced according to an international, rather than a local periodization. This separation of time and space is central to the second element of modernity's dynamism: the disembedding of social institutions. In this, our social institutions such as medicine, education, and culture become separate from local contexts and stripped of specific local orientations. Giddens argues that there are basically two types of 'disembedding mechanisms'. On the one hand are 'symbolic tokens', media of exchange that are of standard value universally. The prime example is money and its circulation through international financial markets. On the other hand are 'expert systems' of technical knowledge.

These systems are held to have international and universal validity. They are of many types, but Giddens make the point that, in our time, the medical doctor and the therapist are as 'central to the expert systems of modernity' as are other more obvious figures such as the scientist and the engineer.

Both these elements of modernity move societies away from systems of social order based on tradition and spiritual authority. In turn, this gives rise to the third element of modernity's dynamism. This involves the profound reflexivity involved in modern culture and modern social organizations. Never before have the members of a society written and spoken so much about themselves as in the modern West. Social scientists of many types provide descriptive and analytical accounts of society, which feed into patterns of social change. Giddens makes the point that this reflexivity has had the effect of continuously undermining systems of meaning and order. He writes:

> In respect both of social and natural scientific knowledge, the reflexivity of modernity turns out to confound the expectations of Enlightenment thought – although it is the very product of that thought. The original progenitors of modern science and philosophy believed themselves to be preparing the way for securely founded knowledge of the social and natural worlds: the claims of reason were due to overcome the dogmas of tradition, offering a sense of certitude in place of the arbitrary character of habit and custom. But the reflexivity of modernity actually undermines the certainty of knowledge, even in the core domains of natural science.
>
> (Giddens 1991: 21)

Ironically, science, as the heir of Descartes' method of doubt, has come to destroy the very sense of certainty that he sought to establish. The absence of a 'non-deceiving' God in the late modern era has meant that self-reflexivity has not led to certitude but to disorder:

> Science depends, not on the inductive accumulation of proofs, but on the methodological principle of doubt. No matter how cherished, and apparently well established, a given scientific tenet may be, it is open to revision – or might have to be discarded altogether – in the light of new ideas or findings. The integral relation between modernity and radical doubt is an issue which, once exposed to view, is not only disturbing to philosophers but is *existentially troubling* for ordinary individuals.
>
> (Giddens 1991: 21)

Whether we characterize the past 20 to 30 years of Western culture as 'late' or 'high' modernity or as 'postmodernity' there are signs that during this period the trend towards meaninglessness which originated in the time of modernity has been ever more powerful and pervasive. The central themes of Enlightenment – the veneration of reason and reflexivity – are seen to have a 'downside', bringing in their wake a lack of any ground or stable order upon which a secure 'way of life' could be based. Thus the alienation identified by Marx in the early modern period is expanded as we move into the era of consumer-centred capitalism and postmodernity.

Postmodern subjectivity

In the last chapter I suggested that with the advent of modernity human subjectivity had become 'pathologically hypertrophied'. On the one hand it appeared to be the 'source of everything', while on the other it was experienced as 'weak and fragile'. We discussed Marx's approach to alienation above. This was connected with the process of production. A number of commentators have linked the rise of postmodernity to a shift in the priorities of capitalist enterprise. Production is no longer the only focus of innovation and development. Consumption is now centre stage. For the continued expansion of capitalism there is both a need for new markets and a never-ending need to incite consumers towards new desires, new needs and thus more purchases. New markets arise not alone from the geographic expansion of capitalism but also from the penetration of selling and consumption into more and more aspects of our lives.[3] One example is the development of childbirth and childhood as arenas in which we can be tutored towards expanded requirements and fashions. Chains of stores with names such as 'Mothercare' and 'The Early Learning Centre' are part of this development. This focus on consumption gives a priority to advertising and marketing. These are concerned with the production and selling of identities and fashions. We are led to think about ourselves in terms of these lifestyles and identities that are presented to us through various forms of media. Increasingly, the narratives through which we think of ourselves and our goals and aspirations are ones given to us by those whose job it is to promote consumption. However, for profits to be made, these narratives require continuous rewriting.

Thus the logic of the current economic system involves an increasing exhortation to consume and to experience our lives in terms of needs to be filled by new products, new services or some new expert discourse. As a result, never before has the realm of internal subjectivity been so well explored. We have books and magazines dedicated to every form of human desire. And yet we experience an even greater emptiness than ever before. The sociologist Nikolas Rose has written about this paradox:

> Consumption requires each individual to choose from among a variety
> of products in response to a repertoire of wants that may be shaped and
> legitimated by advertising and promotion but must be experienced and
> justified as personal desires . . . the modern self is institutionally
> required to construct a life through the exercise of choice from among
> alternatives.
>
> (Rose 1989: 227)

We are, according to Rose, 'obliged to be free'. Not only do we have to
choose items to feed our desires however, but we also have to choose our
values from a range with an ever-decreasing 'shelf-life'. The nihilism of
modernity, as described by Heidegger, becomes an economic necessity in
the age of postmodernity. It is not hidden 'deep' within the culture but
instead is proclaimed loudly from every TV set and billboard. As
mentioned above, Giddens draws attention to the importance of reflexivity in the time of late modernity. He talks about the 'reflexive project of
the self', which he defines as 'the process whereby self-identity is constituted by the reflexive ordering of self-narratives' (Giddens 1991: 244). He
argues, in a formulation that echoes the philosophical analysis of
modernity discussed above, that this process directly leads to an undermining of 'ontological security'. We briefly discussed the writing of Rollo
May above. In his book *The Meaning of Anxiety*, although pointing to the
problem of anxiety as a problem of modernity, May also notes the
powerful 'anxiety-dispelling' effects of the Enlightenment and the advent
of modernity. He notes that:

> The confidence that physical nature and the human body were mathe-
> matically and mechanically controllable had vast anxiety-dispelling
> effects. This was true not only in meeting man's material needs and
> overcoming the actual threats of physical nature but also in freeing the
> human being from 'irrational' fears and anxiety. A way was opened for
> dissolving the multitude of fears of devils, sorcerers, and forms of magic
> which had been the foci of pervasive anxiety in the last two centuries of
> the Middle Ages as well as in the Renaissance itself.
>
> (May 1977: 24)

In other words, the order promised by modernity had the effect of ridding
Western society of many of the fears and worries associated with a world
dominated by spirits and immaterial forces. We have noted the anxiety
associated with the nihilism of modernity above; however, the
Enlightenment promises of reason and individual freedom also held out a
promise of security and of a world under the control of human beings.
Postmodernity robs us of even this promise. The terrors of cultural chaos
and disorder return to haunt us and combine with the ontological anxiety

that is the ongoing legacy of modernity to render postmodernity the true *age of anxiety*.

Ulrich Beck characterized modernity as a 'risk society'. By this he meant that there has been a real increase in the number of threats posed to individuals by science and technology (Beck 1992). However there has also been an increased *focus* on risk, associated with the rise of calculative rationality and reflexivity. In the absence of the moral authority and direction provided by religion, human beings are led to live their lives according to a utilitarian agenda that involves the everyday calculation of opportunity and risk. In a language that echoes Heidegger, Berger et al. (1974) speak about modernity in terms of humanity's 'homelessness' in the absence of 'religious theodicies'. They note that although modernity has achieved many impressive transformations, it has not:

> . . . fundamentally changed the finitude, fragility and mortality of the human condition. What it has accomplished is to seriously weaken those definitions of reality that previously made the human condition easier to bear.
>   (Berger et al. 1974: 166)

It must be said that although the message of modernity seriously under-mined any unquestioning approach to religious faith, it actually gave rise to a number of ideologies that provided alternative frameworks for many people, particularly in the twentieth century. In a number of ways, science, socialism and discourses such as psychoanalysis provided meaningful systems of knowledge, through which people could find a 'moral' order and guidance about appropriate ways to lead their lives. These systems offered a vision of reality in which human progress was a reality. People put their 'faith' in such accounts of our situation and through this achieved some relief from the burden of calculative reflexivity. In the past 20 years anti-foundationalism and post-structuralism have subverted these ideologies and robbed us of 'secure' systems of knowledge about the world and our place within it. In his 1997 book, the sociologist Frank Furedi speaks about our times in terms of a 'culture of fear'. Furedi notes that in the past 20 years Western societies have not only been concerned about risk but also *preoccupied* by it. He points to the paradox whereby the healthier we are the more, it seems, we are obsessed about health. He quotes the study by Skolbekken (1993) of the 'risk epidemic in medical journals'. In this review of medical journals in the UK, Scandinavia and the USA between 1967 and 1991, a phenomenal increase was noted in the number of articles dealing with issues of 'risk'. In the first five years of this period there were just 1000 'risk' articles published, whereas during the last five years there were over 80000. Furedi writes:

> There may be different interpretations concerning the intensity and
> quality of different threats to our safety, but there is a definite, anxious
> consensus that we must all be at risk in one way or another. Being at risk
> is treated as if it has become a permanent condition that exists
> separately from any particular problem. Risks hover over human beings.
> They seem to have an independent existence. That is why we can talk in
> such sweeping terms about the risk of being in school or at work or at
> home. By turning risk into an autonomous, omnipresent force in this
> way, we transform every human experience into a safety situation.
>
> (Furedi 1997: 4)

Postmodernity is thus a time when the established routes through life have
been destroyed and we are left individually to set a course for ourselves.
We are left with fragments of maps, in which we can have little faith. In this
situation the self itself has become the route and while sometimes this is
experienced as liberation, more often, according to the sociologists, it is
felt to be a heavy burden. Our sense of living in a meaningful world is
more fragile than ever and, perhaps, more easily shattered.

My suggestion is that, in so far as PTSD is a disorder that has an
ontological dimension, a concern with the meaningfulness of life itself,
then it is a disorder that we could expect to be associated with the
postmodern era. We saw earlier in Section I that the intrusive-avoidance
symptoms at the heart of PTSD are generally understood to result from the
individual's desperate attempts to make sense of what has happened to
him/her. If my analysis is correct, then PTSD, as a disorder of meaning, is
something that we could reasonably expect to be more prevalent in the
postmodern era and to be an object of concern for the society and its
'healers'. This might explain the increased interest in trauma, discussed in
the Introduction. Before finishing this chapter I would like to point to
other work that has sought to connect other forms of 'psychopathology'
with the culture of modernity/postmodernity. This discussion will not aim
to be comprehensive, but will seek to show how other commentators have
sought to establish the sort of connection under discussion in this work.

Postmodern madness and distress

Psychiatry has long recognized 'culture-bound' syndromes, but these have
usually been patterns of distress located in certain non-Western cultures.
Littlewood and Lipsedge (1986) examine what they call 'the culture-
bound syndromes of the dominant culture'. These are patterns of
dislocation and distress, named and analysed by Western psychiatry as part
of its general nosology but which appear to be particularly associated with
modern Western societies. Traditional culture-bound syndromes are

usually understood to occur in individuals who are relatively powerless and the culturally 'prescribed' syndrome allows the individual to communicate their distress in a way that will be recognized and understood. There is often a triphasic pattern consisting of initial *dislocation* of the individual, followed by an *exaggeration* of this dislocation (this phase involves development of the characteristic 'symptoms' of the syndrome), which is followed in turn by a *restitution* of the individual back into the everyday world (Littlewood and Lipsedge 1986). One example of traditional culture-bound syndromes is 'Koro', which has been described in men in Malaysia, China and other countries in Asia. This involves an intense fear that one's penis is retracting into one's abdomen. The individual takes steps to stop this happening, in the belief that if his penis retracts he will die. Another example, 'Negi Negi', described in young men in the New Guinea Highlands, involves the public destruction of property and the threat of violence. It often occurs in men who are faced with enormous bride-price debts.

Littlewood and Lipsedge make the point that these syndromes do not simply involve the expression of individual distress but articulate 'core structural oppositions' in the society between different groups such as men and women, young and old. They possess a 'public shared meaning' and appeal to beliefs and values that are held in common by members of the society. In his/her display of distress the 'victim' articulates the fundamental (and often unconscious) cultural concerns of the whole community.

When it comes to the 'dominant culture' (by which they mean Western modernity), Littlewood and Lipsedge make the case that syndromes such as anorexia nervosa, hysteria, self-poisoning and agoraphobia (conditions suffered in the main by women), could be regarded as culture-bound. They are infrequently found in traditional, non-Western cultures. They involve the 'inversion' of everyday roles prescribed by Western culture for women. For example, they discuss agoraphobia as 'the housewife's disease' and make the point this syndrome involves an *exaggeration* of the usual woman's social position that is 'in the home' and 'dependent'. In agoraphobia, the woman cannot leave the home and usually an intense reliance on the partner develops. In the case of anorexia nervosa, which is now taking on epidemic proportions in industrialized countries, there is an obvious *exaggeration* of 'normal' slimming and dieting. There is clearly enormous pressure on young women and girls in such countries to control their weight. Attractiveness is often equated in the media with 'a slim figure'. Littlewood and Lipsedge make the point that women are 'more harshly penalized for failure to achieve slenderness as they are more often denied or granted access to social privilege on the basis of physical appearance' (1986: 264).

Giddens also examines the case of anorexia nervosa and argues that a central aspect of this syndrome is the profound degree of 'self-monitoring' involved. As I noted above, a number of writers have drawn attention to the way in which modernity has promoted rational control of the self as an ideal. This control is achieved through regular monitoring and analysis of our thoughts, our moods and our bodies. Giddens argues that modernity has championed the 'cultivation of bodily regimes as a means of reflexively influencing the project of the self'. Anorexia nervosa is a disorder of modernity and can be understood as 'a pathology of reflexive self-control, operating around an axis of self-identity and bodily appearance, in which shame anxiety plays a preponderant role' (Giddens 1991: 105).

Anorexia nervosa appears in the twentieth century and has reached an alarming prevalence in the past 20 years because our culture has, as a central preoccupation, reflexive self-control. Giddens quotes from the therapist Susie Orbach:

> The anorectic woman *encompasses in her symptom a way of being* entirely at odds with the phlegmatic response of her nineteenth-century hysterical sister. Not for her the fainting, falling, or flailing fists; her protest is marked by the achievement of a serious and successful transformation of her body . . .
>
> (Orbach 1986: 27; my italics)

While the epidemiology of anorexia nervosa is clear-cut, and there is little disagreement that it is a syndrome of modernity and postmodernity, the same cannot be said of schizophrenia. However, the psychologist Louis Sass has persuasively made the case that schizophrenia, the central clinical conundrum of the psychiatric enterprise, involves an exaggerated form of self-reflexivity. In his book *Madness and Modernism: Insanity in the Light of Modern Art, Literature, and Thought* (1992b), Sass argues that most twentieth century accounts of schizophrenia have either presented the condition as some sort of 'deficit state' with a breakdown of 'higher cognitive abilities', or as a state of 'wild' abandon, a state of 'Dionysian madness'. The first of these two images is best captured in Emil Kraepelin's original formulation of the condition as *dementia praecox*. This image, allied to the Freudian notion of 'regression' in the work of Eugen Bleuler, has come to shape the dominant approach towards understanding schizophrenia within psychiatry. The condition is held to be caused by some sort of breakdown in mental functioning and the patient is understood to be operating at a 'lower level' or even to have returned to a 'primitive' form of psychological functioning. The second image of madness is more often found in art and literature and even philosophy. This is the image of the 'madman' as wild and free, someone whose desire is not bound by the normal constraints of society. This image can be found in radical psychiatric accounts of madness such as those of R. D. Laing in *The Politics of Experience* (1967) and Deleuze and Guattari's *Anti-Oedipus: Capitalism and Schizophrenia* (1977). Sass points out that:

> The avant-gardists and antipsychiatrists have emphasized the positive side – excesses of passion, vitality, and imagination – yet they, no less than the traditional analysts, assume that the schizophrenic lacks the self-control, awareness of social convention, and reflexivity of 'civilized' consciousness.
>
> (Sass 1992b: 22)

Sass presents a very different interpretation of the schizophrenic experience. He finds strong resonances between the ways in which modern artists and writers have grappled with the contradictions of modernity and the symptoms described by patients who have been diagnosed as schizophrenic. Modern art, according to Sass, struggles with the cultural presence of both alienation and intensified, exaggerated forms of self-consciousness. He says:

> Instead of a spontaneous and naïve involvement – an unquestioning acceptance of the external world, the aesthetic tradition, other human beings, and one's own feelings – both modernism and postmodernism are imbued with hesitation and detachment, a division or doubling in which the ego disengages from normal forms of involvement with nature and society, often taking itself, or its own experiences, as its own object.
>
> (Sass 1992b: 37)

He suggests, in effect, that similar things happen in schizophrenia and explores a great deal of case material in support of this. Sass does not make an argument for a causal connection between modernity and schizophrenia. His work is aimed at helping increase our 'understanding' of the experience of madness, not at producing a scientific 'explanation'. However, he is very much aware of potential objections to his link between modern culture and schizophrenia. Most psychiatrists would object to his work by citing the usual interpretation of the findings of the international WHO studies on the prevalence of schizophrenia. This interpretation points to the similarity in prevalence found in developed and developing societies. Sass takes up this issue in an Epilogue to his book and argues that, by paying attention to the findings relating to onset, course and subtype diagnosis, a very different interpretation of the results of these studies can be made. He makes the case that what these studies do suggest is that the more persistent, and perhaps more prototypical, forms of the illness may well be more common in developed societies. He musters similar support from historical studies of madness in Western countries. While there are obviously no epidemiological studies that one can use to compare prevalence historically, there is evidence that schizophrenia did not appear, to any significant degree at least, until the end of the eighteenth century. This would connect schizophrenia with the birth of the 'modern episteme' that Sass (following Foucault) identifies with the Kantian revolution.

From a somewhat different angle, David Levin (1987) argues in the opening essay of *Pathologies of the Modern Self: Postmodern Studies on Narcissism, Schizophrenia, and Depression* that clinical conditions such as narcissism, schizophrenia and depression are particularly associated with modern and postmodern cultures. His analysis of modernity/postmodernity and its psychopathological effects draws heavily on the critique of nihilism developed in the work of Nietzsche, Adorno and Heidegger. He says:

> I want to draw a clearer, more deeply ontological understanding of the way in which the epidemic psychopathology distinctive of our time is a historical manifestation of a cancerous nihilism: the 'negation' of Being working its slow destruction through the agency of the human will, the human ego. The pathology is pervasive and not limited to a few unfortunates. This understanding of our pathology is what I call my 'ontological hypothesis'.
>
> (Levin 1987: 22–23)

Levin makes a direct connection between the rise of the 'modern self' and the emergence of specific forms of psychopathology. His interpretation of nihilism is not only ontological, he says, but epidemiological. He attempts to demonstrate that some of the 'postures of narcissistic disorders, schizophrenias, and depressions' are 'symptomatically implicit' in the thought of Descartes, with its strong focus on subjectivism. However, these specific forms of psychopathology are merely the 'tip of the iceberg', according to Levin. They are, he says:

> . . . merely the most extreme cases of a collective and archetypal madness – nihilism – at work in all of us. Nihilism is a cultural epidemic that defines the spirit of our epoch. Thus, our cases of psychopathology cannot be understood outside of an ontological field of interpretation in which we acknowledge our present historical experience of Being: our debilitating loss of conviction in the meaningfulness of living; our dreadful encounter with the possibility of nothingness.
>
> (Levin 1987: 26)

These are just some examples of the different idioms – clinical, socio-logical, cultural and philosophical – in which different forms of psychopathology have been associated with modernity. Most of these accounts identify a particular form of alienation, involving meaning-lessness and dislocation, alongside an exaggerated form of self-reflexivity as being involved in the psychological suffering of our times.

We saw in Section I that PTSD, as defined by contemporary psychiatry, is a syndrome that involves meaningfulness and assumptions about the self as central concerns. The intrusive-avoidance symptom complex, which is understood to lie at the heart of PTSD, is conceptualized by many workers as arising directly from a disturbance in the meaningfulness of the patient's world. We have seen above how modern/postmodern culture has been characterized by many thinkers as involving both a fundamental breakdown in the meaningfulness of the world and a particular form of 'pathologically hypertrophied' subjectivity, which renders the self discon-nected and fragile. In bringing these two discourses together my aim is not to develop a new 'causal model' of PTSD. Like Louis Sass, I am not trying to *explain* the causes of PTSD. Rather, I am attempting to develop an understanding of why our concern with this disorder has risen so dramati-cally. In the next two chapters I shall attempt to tease out some of the implications of this. If PTSD is conceived of as a 'disorder of postmodernity' then that could go some way to account for the rise both in the number of cases diagnosed and in the cultural preoccupation with the disorder.

Summary

In this chapter I have made the case that anxiety, understood as a loss of meaningfulness, is not something that is present in all cultures to the same extent. Instead I have argued that this form of anxiety is something partic-ularly associated with the culture of modernity. Furthermore, its presence has become even more apparent as we have moved from modernity to postmodernity. The postmodern condition is one wherein meaning and order are systematically undermined. As PTSD is conceptualized as a disorder in which the victim experiences a profound sense of meaning-lessness and dislocation, I have made a connection between the recent rise in interest in (and possible prevalence of) PTSD and the advent of postmodern culture. My aim has been to support the evidence presented in Section I that the discourse on trauma is not universally valid. My point is that this discourse is itself the product of a particular cultural preoccu-pation with trauma and the sequelae of meaninglessness and dislocation.

It has arisen in Western societies at a time when Western culture has taken a postmodern turn. In the next chapter I will spell out what I think to be the implications of this insight. I will again turn to the later Heidegger to provide a philosophical 'starting point'.

Chapter 10
Responding to postmodernity

Introduction

So far in this book I have used Heidegger's ideas in a number of ways. I have used his concepts of being-in-the-world, worldliness and temporality to highlight the limitations of cognitive approaches in psychology. I have also used these concepts and his account of the ontic–ontological difference to develop an approach to meaning and loss of meaning that situates these phenomena not inside individual minds but in relation to the social and cultural context. In Chapter 8 I introduced Heidegger's approach to technology and his concept of *Gestell*, and I used this as a way of opening up the relationship between anxiety and modernity. Even if we consider Heidegger's account of technology to be overly pessimistic (and many people do, including myself), the fact that elements of his analysis have been echoed widely by other philosophers and sociologists should cause us to reflect on this relationship. We are increasingly aware that there is a high price to be paid for the gains of Enlightenment, modernity and humanism. Human beings have been left 'homeless' and insecure in a world that is increasingly shaped and controlled by them. However we understand the shift to postmodernity it would appear that this has served to make matters worse.

If we accept that human reality is a shared reality and not something simply generated within individual minds then it is reasonable to expect that different social and cultural contexts will produce different ways of thinking about and experiencing emotional states, different sorts of vulnerability and different ways of responding. My suggestion is that contemporary Western, postmodern societies have a particular vulnerability with regard to meaning, order and purpose. The move away from grand narratives has been both a liberation and a curse.

On the basis of this analysis I am suggesting that both the increasing identification of post-traumatic anxiety and our more general cultural concern with trauma can be understood as one way in which this vulnera-

189

bility is manifesting itself. As mentioned in the introduction, I believe that the theme of meaning and its loss is common to other kinds of mental illness as well and has also been raised in relation to suicide, particularly in industrialized countries.[1] The question posed in this chapter and the next is about how we should respond to these concerns. Psychiatry and psychology currently respond through the provision of more technology, mainly in the form of various psychotherapeutic interventions. If the foregoing analysis is valid and our current vulnerability around the issue of meaning is linked to the advent of modernity and postmodernity and the sort of hyper-reflexive subjectivity discussed above, then I believe there is every reason to be cautious about responding in this way. In the next chapter I shall briefly outline current psychiatric interventions for victims of trauma, and discuss the limitations of psychotherapeutic approaches more generally. I develop some ideas about appropriate responses to victims of violence both in Western societies and cross-culturally. In this chapter I want to engage with a more positive aspect of postmodernity: the way in which postmodern thought can help to get us beyond the closed rationality of modernism. This has major implications for work in psychology and psychiatry.

I shall argue that the later Heidegger's writing about *Gestell* and *Gelassenheit* (see below) has served to highlight the dangers of knowledge and the fact that (at certain times) non-intervention and the 'holding back' of knowledge can have positive results. Those arguing for a 'postmodern ethics' have developed this position. In this discussion I shall also look at the writing of Michel Foucault (touched on in the intro-duction) and use this to emphasize the point that deconstructive approaches have an important positive function. By showing that certain assumptions are built into the foundations of dominant discourses, deconstruction works to show that these discourses are limited by the nature of these assumptions. This is a move outside debates about the truth claims of such discourses to a focus on the ever-present mutual dependency of power and knowledge. Through its analysis of the under-lying frameworks of disciplines such as psychiatry, philosophy can have the effect of moving these disciplines from the realm of the necessary to that of the contingent. It does not prove their theories false or their practices wrong but it does render them open to a scrutiny that they usually resist through an appeal to supposedly rock solid (necessary) conceptual foundations. In highlighting the contingent nature of such theories and practices philosophy can also serve to bring into view very different approaches that are usually hidden by the hegemony of dominant positions. While philosophy and sociology cannot tell us what to do clinically, this chapter will go some way towards demonstrating the importance of conceptual analysis for clinical work.[2] In working cross-culturally we move between worlds constructed according to different assumptions, different priorities and different values. In helping us to face this clinical reality squarely this sort of analysis has a *vital* role to play.

Gelassenheit

In Chapter 8, we encountered the Heideggerian concept of 'enframing' (*Gestell*). This was introduced in 'The question concerning technology' and refers to the characteristic form of thought associated with our technological age. Enframing involves an encounter with the world in which everything is experienced as a 'standing reserve', on hand for our use.[3] We saw that for Heidegger this was not just one mode of thought amongst others but also the defining mode in the time of modernity. At its heart is an orientation towards efficiency. In opposition to this, in a number of later works Heidegger proposed another form of thinking. I will loosely refer to this as 'meditative thought'. He called this *Gelassenheit*, in a 1959 book with that title. This has been translated as *Discourse on Thinking* (Heidegger 1966) but the word *Gelassenheit* is usually translated as 'releasement'. In this work he explicitly contrasts the two forms of thought. Calculative thinking is:

> . . . the mark of all thinking that plans and investigates. Such thinking remains calculation even if it neither works with numbers nor uses an adding machine or computer. Calculative thinking computes . . . Calculative thinking is not meditative thinking, not thinking which contemplates the meaning which reigns in everything that is.
>
> (Heidegger 1966: 46)

In contrast, meditative thinking does not attempt any sort of grasping of the world. It is a form of thought which allows things their place. We keep meditative thinking alive by allowing a 'releasement towards things' and by keeping an 'openness to the mystery'. We allow a 'releasement' towards technology, not by fighting against it, or by denying it, but by allowing it its place and by finding in it its own 'mystery'. Heidegger says:

> Releasement toward things and openness to the mystery belong together. They grant us the possibility of dwelling in the world in a totally different way. They promise us a new ground and foundation upon which we can stand and endure in the world of technology without being imperilled by it.
>
> (Heidegger 1966: 55)

Thus, Heidegger does not oppose technology, as such. Through it, albeit in a distorted way, we relate to being. Indeed, in Heidegger's framework we *receive* our technological understanding of being. If we can keep open this idea, of a somewhat passive form of reception, then we have already moved into a non-calculative mode of thought:

> Our technological clearing is the cause of our distress, yet if it were not given to us to encounter things and ourselves as resources, nothing would show up *as* anything at all, and no possibilities of action would make sense. And once we realize – in our practices, of course, not just as a matter of reflection – that we *receive* our technological understanding of being, we have stepped out of the technological understanding of being, for we then see that what is most important in our lives is not subject to efficient enhancement – indeed, the drive to control every-thing is precisely what we do not control.
>
> (Dreyfus 1993: 307)

Thus we have the possibility of moving beyond 'enframing', even though we dwell within it. The difficulty is that we cannot *will* ourselves out of our current dwelling. This was the essential problem for Heidegger: how to keep meditative thinking alive, when it was not something we could consciously grasp at, or aim towards. The picture he paints is of humanity *waiting patiently*. He says:

> If releasement toward things and openness to the mystery awaken within us, then we should arrive at a path that will lead to a new ground and foundation.
>
> (Heidegger 1966: 56)

Famously, Heidegger remarked in his last interview, 'Only a god can save us now.' This remark appears to confirm the idea that passivity is the only option for modern humanity in the face of technological nihilism.[4] When he does advocate particular practices Heidegger points away from any sort of active engagement with the culture or politics of our time. Rather, he talks in terms of a different type of 'dwelling' upon the 'earth', a way of living within the world in a 'non-exploitative' way. We get a hint of what Heidegger is advocating in the lecture 'Building Dwelling Thinking' of 1951. He looks back to a way of life that seems to have incorporated this notion of dwelling. While he is clear that we cannot return there, his tone in this passage is clearly one of reverence:

> Let us think for a while of a farmhouse in the Black Forest, which was built some two hundred years ago by the dwelling of peasants. Here the self-sufficiency of the power to let earth and sky, divinities and mortals

enter *in simple oneness* into things ordered the house. It placed the
farm on the wind-sheltered mountain slope, looking south, among the
meadows close to the spring. It gave it the wide overhanging shingle
roof whose proper slope bears up under the burden of snow, and that,
reaching deep down, shields the chambers against the storms of the
long winter nights. It did not forget the altar corner behind the
community table; it made room in its chamber for the hallowed places
of childbed and the 'tree of the dead' – for that is what they call a coffin
there: the *Totenbaum* – and in this way it designed for the different
generations under one roof their journey through time.

(Heidegger 1993: 361–62)

Many commentators have argued that the thought of the later Heidegger is
simply nostalgic, unhelpful and leads nowhere, or worse, to authoritarian
politics and even fascism. This is the accusation levelled by Habermas in
The Philosophical Discourse of Modernity: Twelve Lectures (1987).
Habermas argues that in his later work Heidegger presents us with a false
and restrictive dichotomy between the all-embracing dominance of *Gestell*
and the passive position of *Gelassenheit*. This analysis of our situation
allows no space for any sort of active politics. We are doomed to 'wait'
while locked in the all-encompassing hold of a calculative rationality.
Habermas condemns Heidegger for collapsing '*all* normative orientation
into the power claims of a subjectivity crazed with self-aggrandizement'
(Habermas 1987: 134). According to Habermas, Heidegger's picture of
Gestell is totalizing and allows no opening for any sort of normative
politics. This leads Habermas, ironically perhaps, to accuse Heidegger of
logocentrism. For Habermas, this means 'neglecting the complexity of
reason effectively in the life-world, and restricting reason to its cognitive-
instrumental dimension' (Habermas, interview in Bernstein 1985: 197).

While not following the critique of Habermas, Miguel de Beistegui
also points to the limitations inherent in Heidegger's later concepts of
technology and *Gestell*. In an attempt to understand Heidegger's
infamous post-war silence on the Holocaust he analyses a number of key
quotations from his works during this period. He quotes the 1949 lecture
titled '*Das Gestell*' ('The En-framing') in which Heidegger discussed the
ever-increasing penetration of the technological approach to life. In the
course of this Heidegger (in)famously said the following:

Agriculture is now a motorized food-industry – in essence, the same as
the manufacturing of corpses in gas chambers and extermination camps,
the same as the blockading and starving of nations, the same as the
manufacture of hydrogen bombs.

(Heidegger, quoted in de Beistegui 1998: 153)

Interestingly, de Beistegui notes that these words do not appear in the published version of the lecture. He points out that there is an unacceptable levelling implied in this quotation. Heidegger seems to be saying that the horror of the Holocaust was somehow 'in the same league' as the problems produced by a 'motorized food-industry'. He appears to say that 'in essence' there is no difference between these happenings. These are all presented as examples of the working out of the logic of *Gestell*. This analysis is not only 'insensitive' but also completely inadequate from any philosophical or ethical viewpoint. The totalizing nature of the *Gestell* allows no position to engage with the evil of the Holocaust as something obviously different from the problems of agriculture:

> When Heidegger defines the enframing as 'the supreme danger' (*die höchste Gefahr*) on the basis of the fact that under its reign man 'himself will have to be taken as standing-reserve', we must wonder whether the death of the victim in the extermination camp does not represent a danger that is other and perhaps greater than the one anticipated in the enframing. Has the victim not moved beyond the status of the standing reserve? Does it not fall outside that logic, outside what Heidegger identifies as the fundamental trait, the essence of our epoch?
>
> (de Beistegui 1998: 156)

De Beistegui also points to the centrality of the *Heim* motif in Heidegger's writings that encounter the political. His discussions of thinking, language and history which remain in thrall to the 'exigency of the return (*Heimkunft*)', and his preoccupation with an image of 'dwelling' which is 'bound to a domestic economy' (1998: 159) are, according to de Beistegui, likely to encounter difficulties in the modern reality of transnational capitalism.

Drawing a positive agenda from *Gelassenheit*

However, a number of commentators have drawn a positive agenda from Heidegger's later writings. John Caputo (1993) points out that these writings have inspired a 'new wave' of Protestant theologians who found in them a much sought-after exit from the existential theology of the post-war years. Heidegger consistently argues the case for a vision of reality that cannot be articulated in material or scientific terms. His concept of meditative thought is easily assimilated to a spiritual quest and he overtly talks about the 'mystery' at the heart of the human situation. Caputo notes that:

> Christian theologians have shown a remarkable interest in and been much nourished by Heidegger's later writings. These writings are

> marked by Heidegger's deeply – albeit generically – religious discourse
> of giving and receiving, grace and graciousness, saving and danger,
> address and response, poverty and openness, end time and new
> beginning, mystery and withdrawal and by a new thematics of the truly
> divine God.
>
> (Caputo 1993: 284)

Heidegger died in 1976. At his funeral, a mass was celebrated by the
Freiburg Catholic theologian, Bernard Welte. Welte (1982) has also argued
for the importance of Heidegger's thought from a theological perspective.
In addition, Michael Zimmerman suggests that the later thought of
Heidegger produces insights that resonate with those produced by Zen
Buddhism. Zimmerman cites evidence that Heidegger was directly influ-
enced by reading works of East Asian religious thought. While Zimmerman
is able to develop a number of similarities between various elements of the
Buddhist tradition and Heideggerian philosophy I wish to quote just one
here:

> . . . both later Heidegger and the Soto Zen master suggest that spiritual
> practices may help put one in the position of a paradoxical 'willingness
> not to will', thereby preparing one for the releasement that brings one
> into the world appropriately for the first time.
>
> (Zimmerman 1993: 256)

Zimmerman also notes how Heidegger's notion of 'letting things be' has
been picked up by a number of thinkers from within the environmentalist
tradition. These thinkers have put forward the notion of *deep ecology*.
They argue for a transformation in the way human beings think about and
encounter their environment, and share with the later Heidegger a deep
opposition to humanist thought. For example, Christopher Manes argues
that deep ecology involves learning a 'new language'. This would involve
removing human reason from its pedestal and developing a position from
which we can 'hear' another language:

> A language free from an obsession with human preeminence and
> reflecting the ontological humility implicit in evolutionary theory,
> ecological science, and postmodern thought, must leap away from the
> rhetoric of humanism we speak today. Perhaps it will draw on the
> ontological egalitarianism of native American or other primal cultures,
> with their attentiveness to place and local processes. Attending to
> ecological knowledge means metaphorically relearning 'the language of
> birds' – the passions, pains, and cryptic intents of the other biological
> communities that surround us and silently interpenetrate our existence.
>
> (Manes 1992: 349)

Thus, the later Heidegger's encounter with modernity has been both an inspiration and the subject of severe criticism. Given his involvement with the Nazis and his post-war silence with regard to the Holocaust, any positive agenda that is seen to rest on Heidegger's work is likely to be the subject of controversy for some time. In spite of this, I believe that his distinction between the *Gestell* and *Gelassenheit* modes of thinking is a helpful starting point. In the next section I discuss how this has had an effect on certain aspects of ethical thought within the continental philosophy tradition. What follows is not meant to be a comprehensive exposition of the emerging discourse of 'postmodern ethics'. I am concerned simply to show how Heidegger's thought has opened up a way of thinking that is of relevance to the encounter between Western psychiatry and other cultures and between psychiatry and critical elements of the emerging service-user movement in Western countries.

While we usually think about technology in terms of such things as factories, washing machines and computers, in my opinion the world of mental health is one of the best examples of how a technological way of thinking has come to take over a part of our lives as human beings. Psychiatric technology is about systems of knowledge and expertise: ways of ordering our reality and our relationships. As we begin the twenty-first century we have a huge (and growing) pharmaceutical industry dedicated to the production of various chemicals to control our thoughts and emotions. Alongside the various psychodynamic therapies we now have cognitive-behavioural therapies and various systems of family intervention. We have numerous 'tools' to assess personality, to appraise motivation and compliance and, of course, to measure something called 'risk'. Psychiatry responds to criticism and crises by asserting its scientific nature and arguing for further research and the development of new tools, therapies and interventions. If even a little of what Heidegger and the others quoted in the last chapter have said is valid then this response is surely part of the problem and not the solution.

'Responsibility for otherness'

Much contemporary ethical theory is, according to Zygmunt Bauman, a product of modernity – a search for rational, universal, foundational ways of understanding the world and determining our place in it. However, as discussed in the last chapter, within the culture of postmodernity, faith in reason, order and science is being undermined, anti-foundationalist philosophies and ideas are coming to the fore. The 'grand narratives' of the past are losing credence.[5] Bauman, who overtly embraces the concept of postmodernity, argues that the modernist search for codification, universality and foundations in the area of ethics was actually destructive of the moral impulse. He argues for a 'morality without ethics'. For Bauman, postmodernity is not about the 'demise of the ethical' or about the 'substitution of aesthetics for ethics', as is often assumed and sometimes proclaimed. Rather, it is about facing up to the real moral dilemmas that face us, without recourse to the illusion that there will always be a rational correct solution. For Bauman, modernity was animated by a belief in 'the possibility of a non-ambivalent, non-aporetic ethical code' (the term *aporia* refers to a contradiction that cannot be overcome, one that results in a conflict that cannot be resolved). He says:

> It is the *disbelief* in such a possibility that is *post*modern . . . The foolproof – universal and unshakably founded – ethical code will never be found; having singed our fingers once too often, we know now what we did not know then, when we embarked on this journey of exploration: that a non-aporetic, non-ambivalent morality, an ethics that is universal and 'objectively founded', is a practical impossibility; perhaps also an *oxymoron*, a contradiction in terms.
>
> (Bauman 1993: 10)

Lyotard makes the point in *The Postmodern Condition* that his analysis of the postmodern provides us with 'the outline of a politics that would respect both the desire for justice and the desire for the unknown' (Lyotard 1984: 67). A postmodern ethics is one that does not shut down possibility and negate difference. In his book *Political Theory and Postmodernism* (1991), Stephen White has clarified some of the ethical issues at stake in the modernism/postmodernism debate. White distinguishes two senses of the concept of responsibility, a key term in ethical discussion. The more familiar is a 'responsibility to act' in the world in ways which are justifiable. He contrasts this with a 'responsibility to otherness' that involves a concern not to silence other voices and thus involves an element of 'withholding' as a central concern. The former is associated with an obligation to acquire reliable knowledge to guide one's actions and is essentially concerned with issues of practical effectiveness. This sense of moral responsibility is most familiar to us because it is firmly attached to the modernist vision. It requires ethical principles firmly grounded in rational analysis and which can be held to be universally valid. This sort of responsibility corresponds to a *Gestell*-like impulse to order and control the world, to make it – and us – function more efficiently and predictably. White links these different aspects of responsibility to different understandings of the nature of language. He says:

> Language can be understood in terms of its *action-coordinating* or its
> *world-disclosing* capacity. These correspond, respectively, to the
> responsibility to act and the responsibility to otherness.
>
> (White 1991: 22–23)

A number of philosophers have put the question of 'action' at the centre of
their systems. These include Anglo-American philosophers such as J.L.
Austin and John Searle who:

> . . . have followed a strategy of analysing how in normal speech, our
> *saying* certain things allows us to *do* certain things (e.g., saying 'I
> promise' under the appropriate or normal conditions also constitutes
> the making of a promise). This capacity of speech acts to coordinate our
> interactions under normal, conventional conditions is what Austin
> called 'illocutionary force'.
>
> (White 1991: 23)

In the development of his speech-act theory, Austin (1980) argued that the
meaning of an utterance depends on the context in which the speech-act
is made. 'Context', in this situation, primarily involves the social conven-
tions that pertain to the act. The success, or failure, of the act depends on
the degree of congruence between the intentions of the speaker and the
actual circumstances or context. A successful speech-act is one where the
correct meaning is conveyed. Derrida, following Heidegger, emphasizes
the 'world-disclosing' dimension of language. He argues that neither the
intention of the speaker nor the context are ever fixed enough that a
speech-act can be judged so simply (Derrida 1988). In the end, there is
never a straightforward 'correct meaning' in any act of communication.
Once an utterance has been made, or a word has been written, it becomes
something that has a degree of independence from the intentions of the
speaker. Communication always involves acts of 'dissemination',
according to Derrida. In addition, he maintains that the context is never
something that is objectively 'given'. Derrida suggests that Austin's theory
privileges a 'normal' usage of language. His arguments are an attempt to
deconstruct this separation of normal from abnormal language and to
show that the conventional conditions for delineating a normal use of
language are hopelessly open-ended and unclear.

In his theory of 'communicative action', Habermas draws on Austin's
work in arguing the case for a 'normal' use of language. In Habermas's
theory speech must be subject to limits:

> These limitations, under which illocutionary acts develop an action-
> coordinating force and release action-relevant consequences, define the
> sphere of normal speech.
>
> (Habermas 1987: 195–96)

In White's view, this leaves Habermas open to Derrida's critique. In the approach to language developed by Austin and Habermas words are basically used by human beings to help solve practical problems and to coordinate the actions of groups of people. For Habermas, the goal of dialogue is consensus. While there is validity in this approach, it is for White, one-sided and partial. If the meanings of speech-acts and written words can never be fully fixed, language is seen to be an open arena of possibilities. It has a dimension that cannot be accounted for in terms of action theory. Sometimes the goal of speech and writing is not consensus at all. For example, poetry is often an attempt to 'stretch' language, to get beyond the conventional givens of what words mean. Language has an 'opening up' dimension, it is what allows a world to be for us. This is where Heidegger's concept of *Gelassenheit* is important. *Gelassenheit* involves a respect for this 'world-disclosive' aspect of language.[6] The 'responsibility to otherness' emerges from both. It involves an openness to the world that is made manifest in a gesture of withholding.

Possibly the clearest account of what a 'responsibility to otherness' would involve is to be found in the work of Foucault. Much of Foucault's work has been concerned to demonstrate the constructed nature of some of our most established assumptions. Our notions such as selfhood, sexuality and reason are shown in his work to be historically contingent 'cultural products'. We do not experience them as such but rather take them as somehow given. Foucault's aim is to show that the order produced in our lives by such givens is not established without cost. As White indicates, Foucault shares with other postmoderns:

> . . . a strong sense of responsibility to expose and track the way our modern cognitive machinery operates to deny the ineradicability of dissonance. The harmony, unity, and clarity promised by this machinery have, for the postmodern, an inevitable cost; and that cost is couched in a language of the Other that is always engendered, devalued, disciplined, and so on, in the infinite search for a more tractable and ordered world.
>
> (White 1991: 20)

Thus emerges the 'responsibility to otherness'. This involves a concern *not* to impose order on the world but instead to allow the emergence of other voices and visions even when this involves increasing complexity and ambivalence. In the three volumes of *The History of Sexuality* Foucault set out to examine how human beings 'problematize' themselves through ethical discourse and practice. His aim was not to put forward an ethical theory, or a new set of values, or to tell us how to achieve our already existing values more efficiently. 'I am not looking for an alternative', said Foucault: instead, 'I would like to do genealogy of problems, of *problematiques*' (Foucault 1983: 231). Such 'problematizations' occur in a culture or an ethos when doubts emerge about axiomatic principles and practices. While Foucault was not about developing an ethical system or theory, he was at pains to promote what Connolly (1993) calls a strong 'ethical sensibility'. In this, Foucault sought to reach 'beyond good and evil' to an ethical position not accommodated within traditional approaches to morality. In much of his work Foucault attempted to track the ways in which power and knowledge were intertwined (Foucault 1977b, 1980, 1981). He argued that the one always implied the other. In this way certain voices in society come to be heard while others are neglected and silenced. In addition, power not only works to silence, it also asserts itself more positively by creating domains of knowledge and discourse. In this process power sometimes manifests itself in a division of the world into good and evil. However, in modern society, which is wary of blunt moral divisions, power more often asserts itself through divisions into true and false, normal and abnormal/pathological. Foucault sought to demonstrate the contingency of such divisions and to deny their necessity. He says that the distinctions good/evil and normal/pathological:

> ... reinforce each other. When a judgement cannot be framed in terms of good and evil, it is stated in terms of normal and abnormal. And when it is necessary to justify this last distinction, it is done in terms of what is good or bad for the individual. These are the expressions that signal the fundamental duality of Western consciousness.
>
> (Foucault 1977b: 230)

The 'ethical sensibility' he worked to develop was about showing the suffering brought about by such regimes. As Connolly puts it:

> Foucault finds a covert problem of evil to be lodged within the conventional politics of good and evil. Evil not as actions by immoral agents who freely transgress the moral law but evil as arbitrary cruelty installed in regular institutional arrangements taken to embody the Law, the Good, or the Normal. Foucault contends ... that systematic cruelty flows regularly from the thoughtlessness of aggressive conventionality, the transcendentalization of contingent identities, and the treatment of good/evil as a duality wired into the intrinsic order of things.
>
> (Connolly 1993: 366)

There are, of course, certain difficulties with this notion of an 'ethical sensibility'. It seems obvious to us that ethics should be orientated towards action, towards the future, towards intervention. A number of commentators have argued that Foucault's refusal to offer a defined set of values that could orientate struggles against domination leads us nowhere. Foucault calls for 'resistance' against domination in a number of his writings, but does not offer a guide to what to put in its place. A typical critique is offered by Fraser, who says:

> Foucault calls in no uncertain terms for resistance to domination. But why? Why is struggle preferable to submission? Why ought domination to be resisted? Only with the introduction of normative notions of some kind could Foucault begin to answer such questions.
>
> (Fraser 1981: 283)

I believe that this type of comment seriously misunderstands the sort of ethics being developed by Foucault. It is not that Foucault has no values to offer; instead he is conscious of the *dangers* involved when philosophers and other intellectuals start to construct ethical systems. He is not in the business of telling us where to go, rather the project is about telling us how we have got to where we are now. He describes his work as a 'philosophical ethos consisting in a critique of what we are saying, thinking, and doing, through a historical ontology of ourselves' (Foucault 1984: 45). What many of his critics miss is the fact that Foucault was very much aware of the power of *his own thought*. In his philosophy it was not possible – and not desirable – to construct a theory which was universally valid. Those who accuse him of failing to do so themselves fail to understand the thrust of his work. For Foucault, the time of the 'traditional' intellectual – i.e. the formulator of universalist theories of human nature and liberation – is past. We are instead in a period where it is important for the intellectual to reflect upon his/her own position and to adopt a more humble approach to his/her knowledge and theories. He refers to such people as 'specific' intellectuals and counts himself among their number. For Foucault, 'the intellectual no longer has to play the role of an adviser. The project, tactics and goals to be adopted are a matter for those who do the fighting' (Foucault 1980: 42).

This does not mean that the intellectual should take a back seat and avoid struggles against injustice or discrimination. Foucault himself supported a number of such struggles. However, he did not want to end up like Sartre, an intellectual to whom people turned for answers, guidance and leadership. Foucault wanted people to question the answers he gave and denied the possibility that someone, somehow could come up with a blueprint for a new society that would hold all the struggles together. He positioned himself as a contrasting figure to post-war communist intellectuals who, arguing from inside a Marxist perspective, could come up with an answer to all political questions and present the 'correct line' for others to follow.

A postmodern ethics is one that is alert to the potential terrors of progress, order and normality. For postmodernists, the modernist and rationalistic attempt to render our moral issues in simple dichotomies of good and bad, right and wrong has had disastrous consequences. For example, Bauman sees such dichotomies operating in the Holocaust. He argues that the Holocaust was not simply an aberration in the development of modern society but instead can be understood as a product of an Enlightenment quest for an orderly society. He writes:

> The unspoken terror permeating our collective memory of the Holocaust . . . is the gnawing suspicion that the Holocaust could be more than an aberration, more than a deviation from an otherwise straight path of progress, more than a cancerous growth on the otherwise healthy body of the civilized society; that, in short, the Holocaust was not an antithesis of modern civilization and everything (or so we like to think) it stands for. We suspect (even if we refuse to admit it) that the Holocaust could merely have uncovered another face of the same modern society whose other, more familiar, face we so admire.
>
> (Bauman 1989: 7)

I believe that there are important lessons to be learned from this by mental health professionals. There are areas of human life that we should not seek to order, because that ordering will have a downside, a set of effects that will not be seen in advance. From the postmodern perspective, the difficulties of institutional psychiatry – such as those described some time ago by Erving Goffman (1971) and more recently in Britain by the Sainsbury Centre (1998) – are not simply an aberration, the consequences of bad behaviour by a few individuals, to be eliminated by new codes of practice and new forms of therapy. From this perspective, they show up as essential aspects of the modernist attempt to control madness and distress. They are its 'other face'. Indeed, from the postmodernist viewpoint the search for ever more efficient therapies and codes of behaviour is part of the problem and can be expected to generate new forms of oppression and suffering.

Summary

The notion of a postmodern ethics does not resolve any of the great problems or dilemmas of modernity. But armed with the 'responsibility to otherness', or a Foucauldian 'ethical sensibility,' we are able to see the world through a different light. We are able to see the downside of modernity, the casualties of progress, the problems hidden from the view of traditional morality. We can experience with greater honesty the immense ambivalence at the heart of our ethical situation as human beings. Bauman says:

> . . . there are problems in human and social life with no good solutions, twisted trajectories that cannot be straightened up, ambivalences that are more than linguistic blunders yelling to be corrected, doubts which cannot be legislated out of existence, moral agonies which no reason-dictated recipes can soothe, let alone cure.
>
> (Bauman 1993: 245)

Postmodern ethics is not about a situation where 'anything goes'. It is rather about facing the world without easy recourse to guiding codes or principles. It is about an acceptance that ambivalence and disorder are here to stay, not just temporary difficulties that need to be overcome by further analysis, or the application of ever more structured ethical systems. Postmodern thinkers would contend that by focusing on the 'responsibility to act', traditional ethics has had to:

> . . . fix or close down parameters of thought and to ignore or homogenize at least some dimensions of specificity or difference among actors. To act in this sense means inevitably closing off sources of possible insight and treating people as alike for the purpose of making consistent and defensible decisions about alternative courses of action. The modern thinker associates the commitment to this sense of responsibility with self-justification either in the sense of moral-uprightness or pragmatic effectiveness. The postmodern thinker, however, sees a deeper, unacknowledged will to mastery at work here.
>
> (White 1991: 21)

Thus, while I concur with philosophers such as Habermas that Heidegger's later work cannot, in itself, lead directly to a progressive political agenda, and while there are profound dangers along some of the paths he has opened up, I do believe that his influence, working through philosophers such as Foucault, has led to important insights about the ethical complexities of our world. In the next chapter I shall bring these insights to bear on the central theme of the book: the question of meaning and its loss and how we should respond.

Chapter 11
Conclusion

Introduction

By now, the reader will be aware that there have been a number of themes running together throughout this book, intertwined in such a way that it is difficult to separate them into distinct subjects or topics. A central concern has been with the question of how our worlds show up as meaningful for us and how this sense of coherence can be lost, particularly in the aftermath of trauma. I have already pointed to some of the implications of this analysis. In this concluding chapter, I want to review the arguments and indicate some ways in which I think we can move forward. From what has been said in the last two chapters, the reader will understand why I shall not be offering a 'new therapy' for PTSD. My analysis is meant to be more of a sort of clearing operation: by questioning the currently dominant approach to meaning and the loss of meaning, I hope to have opened up a space from which new ways of responding might emerge. By stressing the importance of social context I hope to balance what I see as the very one-sided, individualistic understanding of trauma which currently prevails. I have also attempted to show the relevance of Heidegger's philosophy to contemporary concerns in psychiatry. I have used Heidegger not because I think his philosophy holds all the answers but because it confronts us with an alternative account of human reality, one which in turn throws up different ways of thinking about our problems.

In this final chapter, I shall first revisit the major issues of the book and briefly describe current therapeutic responses to trauma, arguing that these are of limited relevance cross-culturally. I then turn to what has been called the 'new cross-cultural psychiatry', in order to develop a positive agenda. The last section involves a discussion of postpsychiatry: the idea that a very different sort of mental health work is possible, one not based on positivism and Cartesian understandings of the self and human reality.

Current discourse on trauma

In Section I of this book, I develop a critical analysis of what I call the 'current discourse on trauma'. This discourse, which has developed around the diagnosis of PTSD, has matured rapidly and now occupies an important and influential position in both psychiatry and clinical psychology. It has been very successful in directing therapeutic attention to a number of suffering individuals who previously had been largely neglected by both psychiatry and society generally. Victims of torture and rape, soldiers affected by their experiences in wartime, children who suffer physical and sexual abuse were all virtually invisible to the gaze of professionals prior to the rise of trauma studies. To this extent, the emergence of a discourse on trauma is to be welcomed. However, in my opinion, the conceptual foundations upon which it has developed have seriously limited discussion of trauma. I suggest that information-processing and cognitive models have become both theoretically and clinically dominant in this area, and that our thinking about trauma is limited by the limits of these models. PTSD is understood to be 'something' discovered by psychiatry and, like other disorders described by medicine, is held to have an objective reality. Furthermore, most PTSD researchers and practitioners assume that it is a disorder which exists, in basically the same form, in different cultures. This has led to the export of the discourse on trauma from Western centres to conflict situations in developing countries.

These assumptions have not gone unchallenged, and I cite as an example the work of the anthropologist Allan Young (1995). Young traces the emergence of ideas about psychological trauma from the nineteenth into the twentieth century, and argues that the concept of PTSD has, in reality, been 'created' (not simply discovered) by psychiatry. In the course of his analysis of PTSD he raises a crucial but little discussed conceptual difficulty that is built into the concept itself. This has to do with the way in which PTSD makes the assumption that symptoms flow unidirectionally from the traumatic event. In a thoughtful analysis of the work of the Australian psychiatrist, A.C. McFarlane, Young raises the possibility that for at least some individuals who have been given a diagnosis of PTSD, a focus on the traumatic event in question is actually the *result*, and not the cause, of other psychiatric symptoms, such as depression and anxiety. This possibility is given added weight by the fact that recent biological research on PTSD would appear to contradict early assumptions that the disorder was simply an exaggeration of the normal response to stress. On the basis of this material, I argue that the sort of causal models that are currently being used in the field of trauma studies are just inadequate to grasp the complex reality of many suffering individuals.

Hermeneutic phenomenology

In Section II of this book, I explore some aspects of hermeneutic phenomenology and how it addresses the key issue of meaning and its loss. I concentrate on the writings of Heidegger as his writing on anxiety is, I believe, of direct relevance to the position I am developing; and I suggest that Heidegger's account of being-in-the-world is more convincing than the Cartesian understanding of human reality. On the basis of this analysis, I argue that the phenomena of meaning and loss of meaning are inadequately accounted for in an empirical scientific idiom alone, and that cognitive approaches to meaning fail to do justice to the complexity of the issue. If one accepts this approach and grants that background intelligibility and meaningfulness are qualitatively different from other 'things', or elements, in the world, then it becomes clear that the ontological dimension of post-traumatic anxiety demands an understanding different from that developed by cognitivism. I argue the case for a hermeneutic encounter with the problem of meaning. Hermeneutics does not seek to grasp background intelligibility in an analytical and scientific way. Instead, meaningful connections are illuminated through interpretations which are never fixed or certain, always tentative and partial.

All hermeneutics is focused on interpretation but Heideggerian hermeneutics argues that meaning is something generated through our practical engagement with the world. We 'know' our world primarily through our practical activities in this world. This form of 'knowing-how' cannot be fully described, or analysed in terms of sets of rules (or schemas) but is the ground upon which our propositional knowledge ('knowing-that') is based. This is an important issue in the context of our discussion of trauma and loss of meaningfulness and we shall return to the implications of this below.

Modernity, postmodernity and loss of meaning

At the end of Section II, I distance myself from the 'universalism' inherent in *Being and Time*'s project of 'fundamental ontology'. Instead, in Section III, I turn to Heidegger's later works to develop my arguments. I position myself against the existentialist presentation of anxiety as a universal mood in *Being and Time* and the associated notion of authenticity as emerging from an individual confrontation (and ultimate acceptance) of anxiety. Instead, I argue that the sort of anxiety described by Heidegger (which does not equate with the everyday psychiatric concept of anxiety, something more akin to Heidegger's understanding of fear) is not universal, but particularly associated with the culture of modernity. In other words, I am suggesting that a sense of meaninglessness, associated with a feeling of dislocation, is something that emerges in a very direct way from the cultural contradictions of modernity. Furthermore, the advent of postmodernity has made these contradictions more acute and robbed us of whatever promises of order modernity could make.

My central thesis is that our current cultural and professional preoccupation with trauma and its sequelae (loss of meaning, shattered assumptions, etc.) stems from a wider cultural difficulty regarding a belief in an ordered and coherent world. I am not suggesting that only people living in the postmodern Western world suffer in the wake of traumatic events. I am arguing that cultures differ with regard to how much 'ontological security' (see Giddens 1991) is systematically put into question. In a society in which the background metaphysics (both articulated and also that contained in the 'way of life') does not function to create a strong sense of life's coherence and continuity, severe trauma or loss can more easily lead to the sort of post-traumatic anxiety described above. Indeed, as discussed in Chapter 1, a similar sort of anxiety can arise without any history of trauma. I believe that many people who end up in contact with psychiatry or psychotherapy are struggling with different manifestations of this kind of anxiety. The corollary is that in other situations, where individuals and communities share an orientation towards life (religious, political or cultural) that gives them a strong sense of coherence, trauma may be experienced differently and result in different sequelae.

Moving beyond interpretation

There is a move in the book from a critique of current (cognitivist) approaches to trauma to the elaboration of a context-centred approach grounded in hermeneutic philosophy. However, in the last chapter I argued that we must also move beyond interpretation and thus hermeneutics. We need to balance these ways of knowing and intervening with insights I broadly label as 'deconstructive'. In Chapter 10, I discussed Heidegger's concept of *Gelassenheit* and the emergence of a 'postmodern ethics'. I used the work of Foucault, Bauman and others to emphasize the idea that a withholding of knowledge can be a positive move. I noted how Stephen White has used the work of Heidegger, Foucault and Derrida to develop the idea of a 'responsibility to otherness'. In my own work with victims of violence in Africa and in Britain (see Chapter 1), I have felt this contradiction between a need to understand and interpret, and an awareness of how dangerous my interpretations and my way of framing problems could be. In the course of three years listening to people in Uganda who had experienced terrible suffering I became convinced that the knowledge I brought with me had little to offer them. Instead, as time went on, I felt that I had more to learn from them about endurance and resilience in the face of extreme tragedy. Individual psychological models, such as PTSD, seemed somehow inappropriate and did not fit with what I was hearing. Somehow it felt wrong to reduce the suffering I encountered – which had historical, cultural, religious, economic and sociological dimensions – to any sort of model at all. And yet many people clearly wanted to talk about what had happened to themselves, their families and their communities during the war years. They were very welcoming and often extremely grateful for my interest and, at times, it 'felt right' to be there, if only to bear witness to what had happened. Thus, there was a need to understand. However, as time went on, I and the other doctor (Joan Giller) working with the Medical Foundation became convinced that we should also hold back from formulating problems in ways learned through our medical training. Joan put it as follows:

> The great danger in projects such as ours is that we actually leave people
> in a more vulnerable position than before, by leading them to believe
> that their ways of coping are somehow inferior to Western ones; that we
> have a knowledge about the effects of trauma on the individual and its
> treatment which supersedes their own knowledge of the ways in which
> healing is brought about.
>
> (Giller 1998: 144)

This tension between a need to witness, interpret and understand and a need to withhold an ordering of another person's experience is not limited to the world of trauma but is present at the heart of psychiatry itself and especially so in its cross-cultural endeavours. In the rest of this chapter I want to outline some possible implications of this analysis. However, I shall begin by briefly discussing the way in which psychiatry responds therapeutically to trauma.

How psychiatry responds to trauma and loss of meaning

From within the current discourse, centred on cognitivism and the diagnosis of PTSD, 'processing' the trauma is essential if the person is going to be able to 'move on'. There is a focus both on the fears and phobias produced by trauma and also on what I have called post-traumatic anxiety and what Janoff-Bulman labels 'disillusionment'. Overcoming fear requires that the victim be helped relive the experience in one way or another and the therapist is required to help the patient face the trauma.

'Processing' also involves work on the patient's beliefs and models, or in cognitivist terms, their schemas. The psychologists Hodgkinson and Stewart write:

> One of the major goals of emotional processing after trauma may be to achieve 'cognitive completion', to integrate the stressful experience with enduring models of the world and one's relation to it . . . The experience of being victimised causes a rupture in the person's personal, family and community identity; if unprocessed, the rupture continues, severing the meaning of all that happened in the past from the present and the future. A continuity needs to be re-established between past and present, and the experience integrated.
>
> (Hodgkinson and Stewart 1991: 21)

A basic assumption in the cognitivist framework is that the meaningful nature of reality is something 'conferred' on it by the schemas, or programs, running in individual minds. Trauma disrupts the meaning of the world through its impact on these schemas. Trauma is thus conceived of as acting on individuals, and therapy is oriented towards restoring or renewing the schemas in discrete individuals. Therapeutic strategies have involved a number of measures aimed at helping the individual adult, or child, to process and assimilate the traumatic experience. Numerous descriptions of these measures are available (see Meichenbaum 1997 for a comprehensive review). With adults, 'cognitive restructuring' is usually performed through talking about the trauma on several occasions. With children, drawing, painting and story-telling are often used with the same aim that the trauma should be relived. This approach has become so widespread that it now appears as 'common sense' to many people living in Western societies. In his book *A War of Nerves*, Ben Shephard quotes the following account from a psychologist working in an American Vietnam Veterans centre:

> In order for a veteran to overcome the paralyzing and destructive effects of his war experiences, he needs to reconsider his Vietnam experiences at three levels: 1. the cognitive or mental, 2. the emotional, and 3. the moral and spiritual. Group therapy with other Vietnam veterans, led by a qualified, caring therapist knowledgeable about PTSD and the nature of the Vietnam war, is often recommended.
>
> In order for healing to begin, the Vietnam veteran needs to 'uncover the trauma'. The specific events which were traumatic to him need to be brought out of repression and into his conscious awareness, then shared in group or individual therapy. There he can be helped to understand the meaning of these events in his life.
>
> (Matsakis, quoted in Shephard 2000: 393)

The trauma, or the traumatic memory, is understood to be 'stuck', or 'repressed' somewhere in the individual's mind. It has to be brought forward, centre-stage, examined and processed. Meaning results from this sort of work. Joseph et al. suggest a conceptual framework for the planning of therapeutic interventions. They argue (1997: 119) that there are several components of the 'adaptation process' and it may be possible to intervene with any, or all, of these:

- promoting re-exposure to the event and to stimuli associated with the event for reappraisal;
- promoting reappraisal of the traumatic experience and its meanings and promoting reappraisal of the emotional states to which appraisals give rise;
- promoting the direct reduction of emotional arousal;
- promoting helpful coping strategies to deal with emotional arousal; and
- promoting the reviewing of previously held cognitive styles and rules for living, some of which may be maintaining symptoms through blocking re-exposure, others of which may determine primary traumatic appraisal.

All of these strategies are focused on the individual and are aimed at making changes on an individual basis. While Joseph et al. discuss the importance of social support, this is very much as an 'additional item'. This is in keeping with other therapeutic approaches. While there is increasing discussion of psychopharmacology targeted at PTSD in the psychiatric literature the dominant mode of treatment is currently psychotherapeutic.

Some therapists argue that this approach can be exported unprob-lematically to different parts of the world. They see trauma counsellors acting like emergency medical personnel: moving rapidly into situations of warfare and other traumas and offering counselling on the spot. Cultural differences are simply ignored. Cognitive and emotional processing can be speeded up using the same techniques anywhere, any time. This position is obviously contradicted by the arguments presented in this book and, in particular, the content of Chapter 4. I do not intend to go over the arguments here. Suffice it to quote from the major report *World Mental Health: Problems and Priorities in Low-Income Countries* (Desjarlais et al. 1995).[1] The authors caution against a singular focus on trauma when helping people who have suffered torture:

> A Cambodian might understand that it is best not to talk about the sorrows of the past, whereas her American therapist might be directed

to help her articulate traumatic events. Indeed, some evidence suggests that detailed inquiries can intensify symptoms. This is particularly true for some refugees from Africa and Southeast Asia, who tend to experience trauma and recovery in ways distinct from the narrative frames of many Western societies, which are often linked to Judaic-Christian notions of catharsis, confession, reparation, and redemption.

(Desjarlais et al. 1995: 130)

An increasing cadre of workers appears to take on board these arguments and acknowledge the importance of culture. However, even among these a majority continue to argue for the importance of Western-type psychological interventions. A good example of this is the call for a 'phased response to psychosocial work' with victims of violence by the psychologist Alastair Ager. He agrees that local cultures are important in determining the ways in which people recover from violent experiences. He also accepts that external agencies should primarily seek to support local networks of social support. However, he maintains that there is still a need for 'targeted therapeutic interventions' because there will always be continuing 'unmet needs'. These interventions should be based on Western psychology:

The delivery of such clinical interventions must clearly take due account of prevailing cultural norms: but . . . it is necessarily and fundamentally driven by external technical understandings of psychological process and function.

(Ager 1997)

Ager maintains that for certain individuals psychological interventions are needed, regardless of culture or social situation. There is still a need for Western expertise. Presumably, he has in mind some form of psychotherapy. In other words, he is arguing for the universal relevance and benefit of this type of intervention. I am not convinced. Ager's position appears to ignore the possibility that psychotherapy can do harm. I believe that therapy can have the effect of increasing the isolation of suffering individuals by encouraging a narrow focus on their own memories, thoughts and beliefs. Such people need, more than anything else, to feel part of a community again, to feel close to other people, to feel at home in the world. Western psychotherapy can have the opposite effect.

To my mind, we face at present the following questions. If the meaningfulness of the world is not given by the structures, schemas or programmes of individual minds but by the practical engagement of human beings with their social and cultural environment, should we look to individual talking as the solution when problems of meaning arise? Is such a framework relevant to cross-cultural work with victims of violence?

Does it help challenge the role of technology and expertise in our society? Are there other ways to respond when the 'magic circle' of meaningfulness is broken? I cannot hope to provide comprehensive answers but some ideas about how we can move forward are already available in the world of cross-cultural psychiatry.

Cross-cultural psychiatry

The relevance of psychotherapy

There is now a considerable body of evidence from the world of medical anthropology which calls into question the universal relevance of individual psychotherapy as practised in Western societies, supporting the conclusion from the Harvard report quoted above. For example, two prominent commentators write:

> . . . the use of 'talk therapy' aimed at altering individual behaviour through the individual's 'insight' into his or her own personality is firmly rooted in a conception of the person as a distinct and independent individual, capable of self-transformation in relative isolation from particular social contexts.
>
> (White and Marsella 1982: 23)

Margaret Lock describes how in Japan, where a very different cultural conception of the self operates, there is little regard for Western style psychotherapy (Lock 1982). In many other non-Western societies different conceptions of the self and its relationship to the social and the supernatural also mean that explorations of inner emotions and conflicts have less relevance than in the West. Kleinman, in a discussion of the Chinese in Taiwan, writes that they invest:

> . . . intimate relationships with more affective significance than one's own thoughts, fantasies, desires and emotions. Family and other close interpersonal relations become a person's paramount interest; coping with them becomes a sign of adult competence, and problems with them are more important to him than other personal problems.
>
> (Kleinman 1980: 134)

Similar considerations emerge with regard to many different non-Western cultures. Although it is a gross over-simplification, Shweder and Bourne's classification of different societies into those which tend towards an 'egocentric' idiom and those which are more 'sociocentric' is useful. With regard to the explanation of illness, in more sociocentric cultures less attention is given to 'intrapsychic' factors and more weight attached to 'independent somatic processes, supernatural forces and social relations as causal agents' (Shweder and Bourne 1982: 111).

In such societies, 'talk-therapy' which aims at relieving symptoms and distress through self-exploration and self-transformation has less validity than in societies where there is a great cultural concern with the individual and the intrapsychic. Christina Zarowsky reports that in her work with Somali people living in Ethiopia there was a great value attached to telling 'emotionally charged stories'. However:

> Among the destitute returnees with whom I worked outside of Dire Dawa, the suffering and narratives which were considered salient were those that indicate – and thus help to create and maintain – an individual's position within the community and its history of dispossession. Attention to personal, private loss or suffering was systematically discouraged, in part, I suggest, because such attention risks causing further fragmentation of moral webs, and ultimately the madness of disconnected individuals.
>
> (Zarowsky 2000: 399)

In the past 20 years, Western 'non-governmental organizations' (NGOs) and the various arms of the United Nations have become increasingly involved with communities in the Third World who have suffered war and violence. Such communities are very often extremely poor and can become dependent on these organizations for health and welfare programmes. Interest in trauma has also emerged in the NGOs and UN agencies involved with victims of violence in Third World settings. There is evidence that these agencies are increasingly 'finding' evidence not of suffering, loss and anger but of 'traumatization' in individuals and communities who have endured wartime violence. They are also in the business of setting up 'projects' to provide counselling and therapy for victims. While these agencies approach their task in somewhat different ways, there is a strong tendency for them to use the discourse on trauma that has emerged around the diagnosis of PTSD. In using this, the trend is for these projects to provide therapeutic interventions that are alien to the local culture and way of life. Furthermore, they often involve a substantial commitment to 'training' and 'education'. This involves local people reconceptualizing their suffering in terms of 'trauma', 'symptoms' and 'therapy'. In other words, a Western, 'technical' way of thinking about suffering and loss is being introduced to people at a time when they are weak and vulnerable. The effect is often to undermine respect for local healers and traditions and ways of coping that are embedded in local ways of life. Based on the arguments developed in this book, I want to make a strong case against these sorts of interventions. I wish to argue, not *against* the provision of support and assistance for people suffering the effects of war, but *for* forms of assistance which work towards an understanding of contextual issues as a priority, and which function from a position of respect for the cultures and cosmologies with which they engage. This position of respect should lead to greater caution with regard to the export of Western psychiatric technologies and 'non-intervention' in certain circumstances.

There are many difficulties in the postmodern position on ethics discussed in the last chapter. However, by dwelling on Heidegger's distinction between the *Gestell* and *Gelassenheit* modes of thought and ways of encountering the world, we can begin to see certain problems in the arena of mental health in a new light. Foucault's 'ethical sensibility', which as we have seen above carries echoes of Heidegger's *Gelassenheit*, can also have the same effect. My interest here is to show their relevance to work with victims of violence in non-Western cultures.

I would reiterate that while philosophy cannot tell us what to do clinically, it can help to clarify what values are being used in the course of certain interventions. It can highlight the assumptions and orientations that normally lie 'below the surface'. With this knowledge we can become sensitive to problems that were previously hidden. As well as attempting to diagnose, analyse, treat and control illness, medicine also needs to develop an awareness of its limits and sensitivity to perspectives other than its own. Foucault's point is that, through simply proclaiming that one has access to 'the truth', one can often be guilty of silencing other, less powerful, voices.

The 'old' and the 'new' in cross-cultural psychiatry

The usual assumption has been that because psychiatry is a 'scientific' discipline, its findings and techniques are, in essence, universally relevant. While culture may superficially influence the ways in which psychiatric disorders present, their basic forms are the same throughout the world. This position has been and continues to be the dominant one in this area. However, it is now regarded by many workers to be seriously flawed and for the past 20 years has been under attack from proponents of what has become known as the 'new cross-cultural psychiatry' (Bracken 1993). (This position has been around for so long now that it is no longer 'new'! Arthur Kleinman introduced the term in a 1977 paper on depression.)

In contrast to the traditional universalism of psychiatry, the 'new cross-cultural psychiatry' has sought to understand the various ways in which madness and distress are represented in different cultures, and to understand the ways in which local people and healers approach these problems in order to comprehend them more fully. From this perspective clinicians and researchers emphasize the importance of understanding the meaning of behaviours and symptoms within local contexts, and apply Western concepts in a tentative fashion only. The 'old cross-cultural psychiatry' continues to assert the adequacy of the traditional medical model while the 'new cross-cultural psychiatry' argues for recognition of the role that other forms of knowledge such as anthropology can play.

The 'old' approach is supported by cross-cultural psychiatrists such as German (1987), Kiev (1972) and Leff (1990). The 'new' psychiatry denies the adequacy of the positivist model (Good and Good 1982). It seeks to show that in many ways our familiar notion of the individual is a purely 'Western' one (Shweder and Bourne 1982) and questions the universality of postulated psychological processes (Marsella 1982; Gaines 1992a, 1992b). The anthropologist and psychiatrist, Professor Roland Littlewood, wrote a comprehensive review of the 'new cross-cultural psychiatry' for the British Journal of Psychiatry in 1990. This is an interesting and valuable summary of the themes and debates in the field. Of interest to our discussion of meaning and trauma is Littlewood's observation:

> It seems likely that the more individualized and Cartesian a particular society's notion of the self (whether as a consequence of industrial- ization, Westernization, or whatever), the more some notion of 'stress' or 'pressure' has then to be introduced to link the individual back to society and to articulate constraints on autonomy.
>
> (Littlewood 1990: 322)

We have already seen that there are three major assumptions contained within traditional psychiatry:

1. a belief in the adequacy of the positivist approach to research
2. a belief that the individual is the appropriate focus of attention from both a research and clinical point of view
3. the assumption that certain psychological processes, because they are biologically determined, are universal.

The 'old cross-cultural psychiatry' incorporates these assumptions. While currently under challenge, the old cross-cultural psychiatry has been the dominant ideology guiding the export of psychiatry from Western centres to hospitals and clinics in the 'developing' world. In an important paper published over 10 years ago in the journal *Social Science and Medicine*, Higginbotham and Marsella gave a good example of how a 'responsibility to otherness' can work in action. By stepping outside the prevailing wisdom and contemplating the possible destructive consequences of the export of psychiatric technology they opened up a different educational agenda that involves a real respect for local ways of life. In their work, they examined the way in which psychiatric care varied little in the capital cities of Southeast Asia, in spite of large social, cultural and linguistic differences between the peoples of these cities. This 'homogenization of psychiatry' was brought about through the inputs of Western (mainly British, American and Dutch) psychiatric experts. Via the mechanisms of international mental health education, consultation and collaboration, a form of psychiatric practice had been created in these different cities that looked to the West for its conceptual foundations and for ideas about innovation and progress. This rendered Third World psychiatry homogenous with:

> [A] common language uniting international and local levels [deriving] from shared assumptions about the shared nature of psychopathology, the use of standardised assessment, and the efficacy of scientifically derived bio-medical or bio-behavioural interventions.
>
> (Higginbotham and Marsella 1988: 553)

While the anticipated effect of these developments was a better standard of patient care, these authors pointed to the unanticipated and very negative consequences which meant, in practice, an actual deterioration in the care received by many people with mental health problems. They stood back from the general approbation associated with the export of psychiatry and presented evidence for serious deleterious 'after-shocks' within local cultural systems. For example:

> The inability of local centres to generate research and evaluate services, in combination with pervasive resource and personnel deficiencies, means that hospitals become custodial end-points for chronic cases. Drugs and electric shock treatment are overused and non-psychotic patients are drawn into hospital work forces.
>
> (Higginbotham and Marsella 1988: 557)

They were able to demonstrate how the diffusion of Western-based knowledge had promoted professional elitism, institutionalized responses to distress and undermined local indigenous healing systems and practices. They argued that, when seen from a perspective located outside the dominant tradition, 'The net result of introducing a formal treatment system for psychological problems is less help for those in need' (Higginbotham and Marsella 1988: 559).

When it comes to the discourse on trauma, which psychiatry presents as being universally valid, we can see very clearly the potential for the negative effects outlined by Higginbotham and Marsella. Thus, there is already a body of Western psychiatrists and psychologists involved in consultation and 'education' in developing countries regarding 'trauma psychology'. This promotes a uniform language centred on the concept of PTSD, treats victims of violence with certain counselling techniques and 'educates' local people in the 'recognition' and 'measurement' of the effects of traumas. The recipients of this knowledge are rendered passive and, in the worst situations, are in fact silenced. Derek Summerfield, who researched NGO 'psychosocial' projects in Rwanda and Bosnia, writes:

> With the world's spotlight on the genocide of April–July 1994 in Rwanda, humanitarian agencies flocked to the region. Soon after the earliest flows of destitute refugees away from the killing, a surprising number of NGOs, some with little knowledge of the country, mobilised psychosocial projects to address mass traumatisation. One of these was a well-known international relief agency whose model – known as Emergency PsychoSocial Care – sought to make an early psychological intervention, both to offer immediate relief and as a preventive measure to thwart the later development of more serious mental problems in the exposed population.
>
> (Summerfield 1996: 14)

With this in mind, as part of their overall strategy, this NGO included an element of 'psychoeducation' for the Rwandan refugee community and produced 75 000 copies of a brochure 'explaining' the symptoms of PTSD. However as there was no word in the indigenous language of the refugees (Kinyarwanda) for the concept of 'stress', difficulties were encountered in the translation process. This did not deter the efforts of the NGO in question and they proceeded to develop a questionnaire and carry out a piece of research:

> First a questionnaire was distributed to evaluate baseline knowledge on trauma so that, after distribution of the brochure, they could repeat the questionnaire to see if there had been 'an increase in knowledge'. The question begged here is: whose knowledge were they talking about, the refugees or the agency's own? The assumption with which they had arrived was that there was a universal trauma response and thus standard knowledge about it.
>
> (Summerfield 1996: 14–15)

This agency went to Rwanda to assist the refugees and help them move forward and beyond the genocidal violence they had suffered. However, their thinking was dominated by a preoccupation with quantification and measurement, and characterized by a faith in scientific psychology and its ability to 'render' the world of the refugees in an 'objective form'. It was assumed that, in this form, the reality of the refugees was available for analysis and intervention. The organization was concerned to be 'active', 'efficient' and orderly. Their vision, I would like to suggest, incorporates many of the features of Heidegger's *Gestell* – the world of the refugees 'shows up' for the NGO workers as something available and 'enframed'. An alternative approach, one aware of the specific historical and cultural grounding of this vision, would be one more in tune with *Gelassenheit*. Such an alternative approach would be able to:

1. recognize the importance of local contextual factors in shaping people's responses to suffering
2. recognize that reconstruction of meaning involves, for the most part, rebuilding a practical way of life
3. work from a position of 'deep respect' for local traditions of healing, local ways of life and local cosmologies
4. work towards an understanding of its own assumptions and orientations, and
5. learn to 'listen' to local voices and learn the skills of what I shall call 'supportive non-intervention'.

This would not abandon the current discourse on trauma but would use it more tentatively and only from a position of deep respect for local situations and ways of life. It would understand the limitations of the PTSD discourse, both because of the particular assumptions on which it is based and also because it has emerged from a society which itself has particular difficulties with issues of meaning. It would pay particular care to understand issues of context while planning an intervention and would make strenuous efforts to 'listen' to local voices and work with local agendas. Summerfield writes:

> The initial aim, surely, is to put ourselves as close as possible to the minds of those affected, to maximise our capacity for accurate empathy and enrich our ways of seeing. It is vital that we do not misunderstand people when they express themselves in their own terms. We want as many as possible of the questions we ask to be right in the sense that they tap what the respondents themselves see as important or urgent.

> (Summerfield 1996: 28)

With regard to the available cross-cultural research on the validity of PTSD, there is no consensus. In their review of 'ethnocultural aspects of PTSD', Marsella et al. write:

> Limitations in the cross-cultural sensitivity of much of the existing ethnocultural research constrains our knowledge about culture-specific aspects of PTSD . . . The measurement of PTSD remains a serious problem because the existing instruments often do not include

indigenous idioms of distress and causal conceptions of PTSD and related disorders.

(Marsella et al. 1996b: 120–21)

On the one hand researchers working from within a strongly medical tradition have, not surprisingly, found PTSD in different parts of the world. However, more anthropologically sophisticated researchers have questioned these findings and have pointed to substantial cross-cultural differences in this area. A recent edition of the journal *Transcultural Psychiatry* was dedicated to the theme of 'Rethinking trauma'. Most of the papers argued for a position broadly in line with what is being suggested here. It is worth quoting the accompanying editorial by Zarowsky and Pedersen (2000) at some length:

> As a general model, however, a highly individualizing view of trauma, which emphasizes catharsis and healing of ethically and politically neutralized 'memories' and 'emotions', is analytically, and often thera-peutically, inadequate, as it risks missing the key themes that converge in the experience of trauma, especially collective trauma. Individuals are always part of overlapping social networks. In the absence of social interaction and a cultural framework, neither emotion nor memory can be meaningfully experienced, expressed or discussed. These social and cultural matrixes are not identical around the world or throughout history. Although culture contact and social change have always occurred and are in many ways accelerated in a globalized economy, nevertheless, not all notions of the suffering self and the links between loss, distress, illness and healing are reducible to the range of 'Western' models, let alone to DSM-IV categories. Indeed, the experience of trauma, war and loss can play a critical role in mobilizing social cohesion and demonstrating resistance as well as resilience.

(Zarowsky and Pedersen 2000: 292)

The reader might ask for examples of a project that has avoided these problems and ask for guidance on how to 'do psychosocial work properly'. This would be to miss the point of my argument. My suggestion is that recovery from violence and trauma is happening all the time as communities rebuild their lives after war. It is in the regaining of an economy, a culture and a sense of community that individuals find a way of living in the wake of terrible suffering.

There are no short cuts. Joan Giller and I left Uganda in 1990, leaving the Medical Foundation project in the hands of a local social worker, Stella Kabaganda. In the years after we left, Stella continued to organize basic medical interventions for women who had been raped in the Luwero Triangle (Giller at al. 1991). I returned in 1995 to see how things had moved on. In a number of villages the women had organized themselves into local associations. They met regularly and had begun to support one another financially through a rotating loan system. This system had allowed them to purchase some livestock and to develop their homes. Some of the local associations had become cultural groups and had written and performed musical plays about the events of the war. At the time of my visit, a new constitution was being planned in Uganda and some of the women had put forward submissions concerning the position of women in Ugandan society. I do not know whether the women discussed their personal suffering or not. The point is that they were primarily concerned to re-establish a way of life. They wanted to move on from the war and wanted to change their social position and that of their children.

My argument is not that the Western discourse on trauma is fallacious or mistaken but that it makes sense only in the context of a particular cultural and moral framework. Its focus upon the intrapsychic, and its proposals for technical solutions are at least meaningful, even if disputed, within a Western framework. However, when exported to Third World or non-Western societies they become confusing and problematic. I would emphasize that I am not questioning the motivation of most of the people who are involved in applying such ideas and techniques. Such workers are confronted by the outrage of violence and suffering in situations of war and seek whatever knowledge is available to guide their responses. However, because of the devastation brought by war, many countries are increasingly dependent on the support of Western NGOs and UN agencies to run health and social welfare programmes. Without sufficient attention being paid to the sort of issues raised here, it is likely that a great deal of damage can be done.

Responding to meaninglessness in a postmodern context

Apart from questions about the export of the discourse on trauma from the West to the developing world, the analysis presented in this book also raises issues about how we respond to trauma and loss of meaning in a Western context. As we have seen above, the standard approach is from within psychiatry and involves some sort of 'cognitive and emotional processing' of the traumatic event(s). If the reader is convinced by the critique of cognitivism developed in this book and its location of meaning and its loss within individual minds, then he/she will understand my concern to explore alternative ways of engaging with these issues. In addition, if the reader accepts (even partially) the Heideggerian understanding of technology and modernity discussed above then the severe shortcomings of framing problems of meaning in a technical (psychological or medical) idiom become apparent. If my analysis is valid then technology itself is implicated in our vulnerability to such problems. We should be wary of turning to it for solutions.

In spite of this there is evidence that psychiatry is everywhere attempting to make itself more technological. The recent 'decade of the brain' and the rise of biological psychiatry in the past 20 years is testimony to this. Psychopharmacology is currently the principal way of responding to distress, dislocation and madness and most psychiatric research is based on a biological paradigm. Since the introduction of the *DSM III* in 1980 (see Chapter 2), a great deal of energy has been spent on the 'science' of psychiatric classification.[2] More and more aspects of our lives have been formulated in terms of mental illness. Over 300 different mental illnesses are now described by the DSM, the majority 'identified' in the past 20 years. In a recent critical account of this expansion, Kutchins and Kirk write that:

> DSM is a guidebook that tells us how we should think about manifestations of sadness and anxiety, sexual activities, alcohol and substance abuse, and many other behaviours. Consequently, the categories created for DSM reorient our thinking about important social matters and affect our social institutions.
>
> (Kutchins and Kirk 1999: 11)

Increasingly, psychiatric thinking and technology penetrate ever further into our lives and our relationships. Alongside drugs and diagnosis, we have numerous forms of therapy to deal with our hurts and losses. We have technologies of family intervention and numerous instruments to assess everything from risk to religious beliefs. Are these developments inevitable? Should we, could we, seek to control them?

In the last chapter we saw how Habermas criticized Heidegger's understanding of technology as 'totalizing'. If every aspect of our lives is structured by technology, and if there is no escape, then according to Habermas, there is no space for a democratic politics. While I am sympathetic to Heidegger's position I agree with Habermas on this point. I don't think we can simply abandon the technologies we have developed to understand and treat states of madness and distress. However, we do need to open up these approaches to debate and examine other possibilities. In his book *Questioning Technology* (1999), Andrew Feenberg discusses this debate about technology at some length. He writes:

> Real change will come not when we turn away from technology toward meaning, but when we recognize the nature of our subordinate position in the technical systems that enrol us, and begin to intervene in the design process in the defence of the conditions of a meaningful life and a lovable environment.
>
> (Feenberg 1999: xiv)

When it comes to the world of what we call mental illness, I am not arguing that we should abandon psychotherapy or psychopharmacology. What I am seeking is a democratic debate about the nature of these interventions: the values that guide them, the philosophical assumptions upon which they were developed and which continue to sustain them and the practical priorities they give rise to. To have this debate we need to be aware of the wider implications of the turn towards a technological idiom. These issues cannot be decided within the pages of professional journals. They are not about the short-term efficacy of one technique or another but about the implications for all of us of a move to frame our difficulties in a particular way.

As I write, in Western Europe we are witnessing a substantial expansion of organic forms of agriculture. This shift is driven not by a concern to reduce costs or to increase efficiency but rather by a different set of values and priorities from those dominant in European agriculture throughout the twentieth century. Organic farmers do not reject the sciences of biology or agriculture but instead want to use the insights of these sciences within the framework of a different ethical relationship between human beings, farm animals and the natural environment. I don't want to stretch the analogy too far: I am certainly not advocating a more 'organic' psychiatry! However, I do believe that we can learn from these developments, and in particular the way in which scientific expertise is not rejected by proponents of the organic movement, but placed in a different position relative to ethical, social and political considerations. This new form of agriculture holds on to elements of modernism but also looks back to pre-modern modes of farming and ahead to patterns of animal rearing and cultivation which take on board global concerns about the environment and the general state of our planet.

Similar debates have long been a part of psychiatry, which has never really sat comfortably within the embrace of modernism. I will end the book by mentioning the notion of 'postpsychiatry', an idea developed by myself and my colleague Phil Thomas in recent years (Bracken and Thomas 2001). This represents our attempt to think beyond a technological agenda for mental health, an attempt to foreground issues of ethics and values.

Postpsychiatry

The idea of postpsychiatry is an attempt to think beyond the theory and practice of psychiatry as developed in the twentieth century. It accepts the Foucauldian premise that psychiatry was very much a child of the European Enlightenment and its focus on reason and the individual self. It argues that psychiatry in the last century merely extended this agenda and worked to silence alternatives. This position has already been elaborated in Chapter 2. By the term 'postpsychiatry' we are seeking to get beyond the old debates between psychiatry and anti-psychiatry. The latter sought to show that psychiatry was repressive and based on a mistaken medical ideology. Anti-psychiatrists wanted to liberate mental patients from its clutches (Bracken 1995). Psychiatry reacted defensively to this and asserted that its opponents were simply 'driven by ideology' (Roth and Kroll 1986). Both sides approached madness as something to be accounted for, something to be written about and something for which therapy was needed. There was an assumption that the truth could, and should, be spoken about states of madness and distress. Both sides of the argument assumed that truth and ideology were mutually exclusive.

Unlike anti-psychiatry and previous forms of critical psychiatry (Ingleby 1980, Kovel 1988), postpsychiatry does not itself propose new theories about madness but by a deconstruction of psychiatry seeks to open up spaces in which other, alternative, understandings of madness can assume a validity denied them by psychiatry. This is the philosophy behind this current work. I have not attempted to develop a new theory or therapeutics of trauma or PTSD. Similarly, postpsychiatry seeks to distance itself from the therapeutic implications of anti-psychiatry. It does not propose any new form of therapy to replace the medical techniques of psychiatry. Anti-psychiatry, especially as developed by R. D. Laing, proposed a modified version of psychoanalysis (based largely on existential philosophy) as an alternative to psychiatry. Both Ingleby and Kovel also looked to different versions of psychoanalysis to frame their theories and practice. As should be clear to the reader by now, I do not consider Freudian psychoanalysis (or even the daseinanalysis of Boss and Heidegger) to be the solution to our current difficulties. I am seeking not only a contextualist understanding of madness and distress but also to open up ways of helping which engage directly with aspects of the social context whenever this is possible. If I can use a spatial metaphor, postpsychiatry is not a place, a set of fixed ideas and beliefs. Instead, it is more like a set of orientations that together can help us move on from where we are now. It does not seek to prescribe an endpoint and does not argue that there are 'right' and 'wrong' ways of tackling madness.

The term 'postpsychiatry' obviously echoes other postmodernist arguments and debates and is particularly influenced by the sort of postmodern ethics discussed in the last chapter. I do not believe that a postmodernist perspective undermines the validity of other critical perspectives such as those derived from Marxist theory. In fact, I am sympathetic to the position of writers such as Jameson (1991) and Harvey (1989) who seek to understand the *culture* of postmodernity in terms of underlying transformations in the nature of capitalism. Jameson speaks of postmodernity as the 'cultural logic of late capitalism', while Harvey sees it as emerging from a new 'flexible form of capital accumulation'. I am seeking to work with insights derived from postmodern theory to develop a *theoretical* framework that can support radical change in the area of mental health. However, I concur with Parker (1998) that there are dangers inherent in the postmodernist position. In the end, theory should serve practice, not the other way around, and our main task now is the transformation of mental health care.[3]

A mental health practice influenced by a postpsychiatry philosophy would work with the following sort of priorities:

1. A foregrounding of ethical issues
2. A move towards contextualist understanding and practice
3. A recognition of power differentials.

These are discussed in more detail below.

Foregrounding ethical issues

Just as the organic movement in agriculture attempts a practice of farming which is based on a new ethical relationship between farmers, consumers, animals and the natural environment, so too postpsychiatry seeks to establish a practice that is centred on a concern with dignity and respect. Medical science is not seen as the final arbiter of what shall count as evidence of good practice. Instead questions of values are put first and ways of helping are pursued which stem from these. This priority of values over science is not new. Indeed, it is clear that the people who argued against the physical restraint of mental patients in the early part of the nineteenth century did so for *moral*, not medical or scientific reasons. The Retreat, set up by the Tuke family in York in 1796, was based on a strong ethical perspective on the care of the mentally ill. Roy Porter in his book on the history of medicine writes:

> The Retreat was modelled on the ideal of family life, and restraint was negligible. Patients and staff lived, worked and dined together in an environment where recovery was encouraged through praise and blame, rewards and punishment, the goal being the restoration of self-control. The root cause of insanity, physical or mental, mattered little. Though far from hostile to doctors, the Tukes, who were tea merchants by profession, stated that experience showed nothing medicine had to offer did any good.
>
> (Porter 1997: 498)

The reforms introduced by the Tukes over 200 years ago were successful and many doctors incorporated their ideas in later service developments. The point is that that the impetus for change came not from the developments of medical science or new breakthroughs in the medical understanding of madness but from an ethical outrage at the way in which fellow human beings were being treated and made to suffer. Knowledge is never free from values and political intent. All knowledge emerges from a position of interest. Psychiatry has sought to present itself as being based upon a disinterested scientific account of madness and distress. However, postpsychiatry accepts that an ethic of social exclusion has been built into the heart of the psychiatric enterprise. Psychiatry is premised upon the assumption that reason has a right – indeed, a duty – to speak about madness. Psychiatry assumes that it is justified in its own attempt to describe, analyse and, ultimately, diagnose madness. Postpsychiatry believes that these are ethical assumptions that cry out to be exposed. Postpsychiatry seeks to begin with values and a debate about ethics and argues that the use of knowledge and technology should be a secondary event. Postpsychiatry seeks to end the monologue of reason about madness and opens up a space where a positive value of madness can be revealed.

Moving towards contextualist understanding and practice

This theme is central to what has gone before in this book. We saw in Chapter 2 how psychiatry has systematically sought to frame its understandings in positivist and individualist terms. This position downplays the importance of contextual issues. I argued in Chapter 2 that one of the most influential books in twentieth century psychiatry was Karl Jaspers' *General Psychopathology* (1963). Contemporary biological, behavioural and cognitivist approaches use a descriptive vocabulary largely derived from Jaspers. The other great influence on twentieth century psychiatry was Freudian psychoanalysis. The language of psychodynamics is also widespread in contemporary mental health practice. In the position being argued for here, both Husserlian phenomenology and Freudian psychoanalysis are discourses that locate the mental arena 'inside heads' (Henningsen and Kirmayer 2000). In this book I have tried to derive from Heidegger and others an approach that is not 'internalist' or reductionist.

The approach to trauma presented here could also be used with other problems encountered by psychiatry. I have mentioned the work of Louis Sass at a number of points in the book. Sass argues that psychotic experience is inherently bound up with the social and cultural milieu of the person in question. Similarly, the essays in the book *Culture and Depression* edited by Kleinman and Good (1985) present depression as variable and socially and culturally embedded.

Recognition of power differentials

The focus of this book is the question of trauma. My aim is to open a space in which genuine dialogue can begin to unfold, a space in which psychiatry has a role, but only alongside other forms of knowledge and understanding. Most importantly, this is a space characterized by a respect for alternative sets of priorities, ways of support which do not involve notions of mental health or mental illness and forms of healing not based in the various forms of dualism built into Western understandings. I have quoted the work of Arthur Kleinman at a number of points in this work. Kleinman is Professor of Psychiatry and Anthropology at Harvard. In his book *Rethinking Psychiatry: From Cultural Category to Personal Experience* he argues for a substantial rethink of psychiatry's agenda. Kleinman criticizes the 'positivist bias' of psychiatry and argues the case for a substantial role for other disciplines. In particular, he suggests that:

> Cross-cultural comparison, appropriately applied, can challenge the hubris in bureaucratically motivated attempts to medicalize the human condition. It can make us sensitive to the potential abuses of psychiatric labels. It encourages humility in the face of alternative cultural formulations of the same problems that are viewed not as evidence of the ignorance of laymen, but as distinctive modes of thinking about life's troubles. And it can create in the psychiatrist a sense of being uncomfortable with mechanical application of all too often taken-for-granted professional categories and the tacit 'interests' they represent'
>
> (Kleinman 1988: 17)

Postpsychiatry seeks to open up such discussions and dialogues in areas other than the cross-cultural. Psychiatry has already been challenged to move in this direction. Philosophy has a substantial role to play here. My approach has been to use insights from within the continental philosophy tradition to open up the assumptions of psychiatry for examination.

However, there is also an important and ever expanding critical literature which draws on the analytic philosophy tradition. Fulford (1994) has used the linguistic analytical approach to highlight the prevalence of, and significance of, value judgements within psychiatric classifications (see Chapter 1). In an approach to mental illness that identifies the centrality of issues of value, the patient's account of his/her own position becomes central. An increasingly important 'user movement' (made up of patients, ex-patients and their supporters) has emerged in different parts of the world in recent years.[4] This movement has begun to challenge some of the fundamental assumptions of psychiatry and has argued the case for forms of support and assistance in times of crisis that owe little to traditional psychiatric theory or practice. For example, the Hearing Voices Network[5] is a loose organization of people who hear voices. Some have received psychiatric care, others have not. They oppose the psychiatric orthodoxy that the experience of hearing voices is always best characterized in terms of auditory hallucinations, i.e. as being a symptom of mental illness. They argue for the validity of other forms of explanation including spiritual and other supernatural accounts. They do not oppose psychiatry as such (and many members of the network take psychiatric medication), but they do oppose the dominance of psychiatric perspectives and its limited understanding of human reality. Similar networks are beginning to emerge in relation to other experiences and behaviours as well: for example, a national network of people who 'self-harm' has been developing in Britain. Peter Campbell argues that the concept of 'crisis' needs substantial rethinking:

> Sadly, I am convinced that for many mental health workers it remains true that they do not think the content of our crises, particularly those they define as psychotic, are real, relevant or of anything but negative value. It is ironic that while increasing numbers of people in the user/survivor movement are seeking new meanings in their most vivid personal experiences, so many mental health workers continue to look the other way.
>
> (Campbell 1996: 182)

A narrow positivist approach to research and theory building cannot hope to cope with these demands and developments, which involve questions of values and ethics, and debates about the nature of madness. In the same way that cross-cultural psychiatry requires a deep respect for other realities, so too the recipients of psychiatry are claiming respect for their own realities. Both demand to be heard in their own words and should not be silenced by the powerful voice of psychiatry.

Endnotes

Chapter 1

1. This work has led to the recent publication of a book on the subject of wartime violence and its psychological effects: see Bracken and Petty (1998) *Rethinking the Trauma of War*.
2. I would recommend the recent biography of Heidegger by Rüdiger Safranski, *Martin Heidegger, Between Good and Evil* (1998), for a full discussion of these issues.
3. See the essay 'Phenomenology, psychology, and science' by Keith Hoeller (1988) for an excellent discussion of the relationship between Heideggerian phenomenology and scientific psychology.
4. The term phenomenology is often used in psychiatry to indicate a listing of symptoms that correspond to a particular disorder. Thus one hears discussions of the 'phenomenology of depression' and other conditions. Phenomenology, in this sense, is simply about the description of various abnormal mental states. In the wider world of philosophy the term is used somewhat differently. It refers to a movement within continental philosophy that sought an alternative to all reductionist accounts of human consciousness.
5. While difficult to define precisely, the word hermeneutics is usually taken to mean something like 'the art or theory of interpretation' (Cambridge Dictionary of Philosophy 1995). As Phillips notes, the word is derived 'from the Greek verb *hermeneuein*, which means "to interpret", and the noun *hermeneia*, "interpretation" (and both associated with the god Hermes, who was a messenger)' (Phillips 1996: 61). In this book I shall use the term to refer to any approach to human reality which emphasizes the meaningful nature of human life and which stresses the importance of interpreting human beings and their actions by way of reference to the contexts in which they live. Hermeneutic approaches stress the *primacy* of this meaningful level of human reality and deny that it can be reduced to explanation in terms of other elements. While hermeneutic philosophy has traditionally been seen as an element of 'continental philosophy', more recently a number of analytic philosophers have embraced the term, most famously Richard Rorty in his influential *Philosophy and the Mirror of Nature* (1979).
6. For example, see Bracken (2001): 'Postpsychiatry in action: the radical possibilities of Home Treatment.'

Chapter 2

1. My discussion of the Enlightenment cannot hope to be comprehensive. In this chapter I am seeking to identify the way in which psychiatry only became a possibility within a cultural context shaped by Enlightenment concerns with reason and interiority. However, I am aware that the positivism embraced by psychiatry reflected only one strand of Enlightenment thought. My account is therefore partial. For example, I do not discuss the importance attached to historical context in the thought of philosophers such as Montesquieu, Hume, Herder and Hegel. One thing is agreed by all students of the movement: the Enlightenment involved a dramatic reorientation of intellectual life, it meant looking to the future rather than the past, and finding in reason itself the path to this future. In this venture philosophy was to have a vital role, for it was through a critical philosophy that both the potential and the limits of reason could be defined.

2. *Cogito ergo sum*: 'I am thinking, therefore I exist.'

3. The word transcendence refers to the property of being outside, or (figuratively) above, other things. In philosophy, something is transcendental if it is of a higher order: 'a transcendental argument . . . is one that proceeds from premises about the way in which experience is possible to conclusions about what must be true of any experienced world' (Cambridge Dictionary of Philosophy 1995: 807).

4. It should be noted that the philosopher Dagfinn Follesdal argues that Husserl moved away from a Cartesian perspective in a number of works and suggests that his philosophy was closer to Heidegger than is often understood. He has engaged in a debate about this issue with Hubert Dreyfus over a number of years (Follesdal 2000). As stated previously, my approach to this debate is greatly influenced by Dreyfus. In reply to a recent piece by Follesdal in which there are a number of quotations from Husserl suggesting a less Cartesian orientation, Dreyfus writes:

   > Husserl often comes up with phenomenological observations that might well have inspired Heidegger or Merleau-Ponty, only to distort them to fit into his account of the constitutive role of transcendental subjectivity.
   >
   > (Dreyfus 2000: 334)

   For the purposes of this book I will stick with Dreyfus and take it as granted that Husserl was indeed following in the footsteps of Descartes. What is important here is Husserl's influence on psychiatry.

5. We have seen above how Descartes put an emphasis on the intellect and looked to mathematics to guide progress. He and other philosophers who endorsed this focus on reason became known as rationalists. Scientists and philosophers who put the emphasis on the importance of objective observation were known as empiricists.

6. In the scholastic period Aristotle was simply known as 'the philosopher'.

7. This was published in six volumes between 1830 and 1842. It contains an encyclopaedic account of the sciences. It expounds positivism and introduces the discipline of sociology.

8. To some extent the naturalist perspective is already incorporated in Polkinghorne's definition of positivism through the rejection of metaphysics.

9. I will not discuss here the differences between 'logical positivism' and 'logical empiricism', nor the differences between 'phenomenalism' and 'physicalism'. For the purposes of my explication of psychiatry's underlying philosophical systems the two central elements of the positivist framework are its prescriptions about the collection of data and about the construction of theories.

10. In fact positivism extends far beyond biological psychiatry. Most social psychiatry in the twentieth century was a search to identify social 'factors' implicated in mental illness and the development of causal theories to account for these effects. A classic example is the work of Brown and Harris. See their *Social Origins of Depression: A Study of Psychiatric Disorder in Women* (1978).

11. A position within philosophy of mind that argues that there is no such thing as mental phenomena as such. Philosophers of this school believe that science will eventually eliminate the need for our everyday language of mental states ('folk psychology').

12. In a 1994 paper in the journal *Philosophy, Psychiatry, and Psychology* Dan Lloyd did make some tentative remarks about a connectionist approach to trauma in the context of an attempt to produce a network model of a Freudian case study.

13. See for example Dreyfus (1994): *What Computers Still Can't Do: A Critique of Artificial Reason.*

Chapter 3

1. Friedman and Marsella (1996: 15) note: 'Criterion B, the *intrusive recollection* criterion, includes symptoms that are perhaps the most distinctive and readily identifiable symptoms of PTSD.'

2. This early Freudian belief in the importance of 'facing up to the trauma' resonates with the sentiments quoted from Kilpatrick, above, with regard to the importance of challenging 'avoidance behaviour'.

Chapter 4

1. This effect of rioting on mental health has also been observed in the USA; see Fogelson (1970) and Greenley et al. (1975).

2. We noted above that somatic symptoms were the most commonly described mode of distress in soldiers in both the First and Second World Wars.

3. In *DSM IV* the various criteria used for making a diagnosis of PTSD are labelled A, B, C, D and E. Thus, criterion A concerns the fact that the diagnosis can only be made if the person has experienced a severe trauma. Criterion B relates to *intrusive recollection* symptoms, criterion C to *avoidant/numbing* symptoms and criterion D to *hyperarousal* symptoms. Criterion E relates to time scales.

4. See, for example, the review by Krystal et al. (1989).

Chapter 5

1. The word 'embodiment' is used in this work in an attempt to get across the idea that we *are* our bodies. This is in contrast to the more Cartesian connotations of *having a body*. Thomas Csordas says that the body is the 'existential ground of culture and the self' (Csordas 1994).

2. In the introduction, I pointed out that Heidegger himself was at pains to distance himself from cultural theory. As I shall show below he presented his account of experience as something that was universal. He did not consider his work to be 'anthropological' in any sense. However, there is now a substantial literature that brings together hermeneutic philosophy with anthropological enquiry: see, for example, Bernstein (1983) *Beyond Objectivism and Relativism: Science, Hermeneutics and Praxis*. In this work I am broadly following the interpretation of Heidegger developed by Hubert Dreyfus (1991). He writes that 'Heidegger follows Wilhelm Dilthey in emphasizing that the meaning and organization of a culture must be taken as the basic given in the social sciences and philosophy and cannot be traced back to the activity of individual subjects' (1991: 7). This is the sense in which I use the notion of human beings as always 'culturally situated'. I will comment again on Dilthey's influence on Heidegger in Chapter 8.

3. The implications of this for cross-cultural work with victims of violence are spelt out in Chapter 11.

4. McCall (1983) indicates that no acceptable English translation of *Dasein* has been agreed on. A literal translation would be 'to be there' or 'being there'. *Dasein* in colloquial German can mean 'everyday human existence' (Dreyfus 1991: 13) and Heidegger is clearly referring to human reality when he uses the term. However, *Dasein* means something more than simply 'conscious subjectivity'. Heidegger is striving to get away from a view of human reality as something grounded in a meaning-giving transcendental subject. As we have already seen such a view has dominated Western thought from Descartes through Kant to the work of Husserl. He says:

> One of our first tasks will be to prove that if we posit an 'I' or subject as that which is proximally given, we shall completely miss the phenomenal content (Bestand) of Dasein.
>
> (Heidegger 1962: 72)

So *Dasein* is not the personal self. While it does have a quality of mineness (see Heidegger 1962: 68) it is apparent that Heidegger is trying to move beyond an atomistic vision of human reality. This is an important issue because many in the existentialist psychiatry and psychotherapy school appear to have mistakenly interpreted Dasein as being an autonomous individual subject. This has led to a type of individualism that imbues many forms of existentialist therapy. In the next chapter I shall mention Heidegger's critique of the work of Ludwig Binswanger, which centred on this issue. McCall opts to translate the term as 'being present' or 'human presence'. However, 'being present' is problematic given the importance in Heidegger's work of the concept of *Vorhandenheit*, which is usually translated as 'present-at-hand'. Emmanuel Levinas (1978) uses the French term '*l'existant*', 'the existent', and Dreyfus simply uses the term 'human being'. For the most part I shall stick to Heidegger's own term – Dasein – and occasionally, when an English equivalent is needed, follow Dreyfus and use the term 'human being'.

5. Sass notes that both Kant and Husserl also made this criticism of Descartes but according to Heidegger neither was able to liberate himself completely from this tendency to treat human subjectivity ontically. Thus, according to Heidegger, both Kant and Husserl tend to portray the transcendental subject as if it could, in princi-

ple at least, be separated from the world around it. This is the result of treating the subject and world as two objects existing alongside within the world.

6. In the next chapter I will discuss some of Heidegger's own thoughts on the subject of 'bodyhood', as presented in the *Zollikon Seminars*.

7. This is similar to the position taken by Rorty (1979, 1980).

8. Within modernity this extemporal vantage point has been associated with the search for certainty and the emergence of the 'transcendental pretence' discussed in Chapter 2.

Chapter 6

1. Safranski notes that Heidegger suffered a 'physical and mental breakdown' in 1946 and underwent a course of 'psychosomatic treatment' by von Gebsattel, a follower of Binswanger. Apparently Heidegger said of his treatment: 'And what did he do? He took me on a hike up through the forest in the snow. That was all. But he showed me human warmth and friendship. Three weeks later I came back a healthy man again' (Safranski 1998: 351–52).

2. These seminars took place at Boss's home in Zollikon, near Zurich, up to three times each semester during this period. Boss published transcripts of these teaching sessions in German (*Zollikoner Seminare*, published by Klostermann) in 1987. At the time of writing, two translated extracts were available: Boss (1988a) and Heidegger (1988). In addition, Richardson (1993) and Dallmayr (1991: 211–37) provided English language readers with accounts of the seminars. My account is based on these English language works. Since the manuscript went to the publishers a translation of the book edited by Boss has appeared, see Heidegger (2001)

3. Heidegger's orientation is basically the same as that in *Being and Time*, which goes some way to demonstrate that the separation of his work into 'early' and 'late' is somewhat artificial, even though I shall make use of it in Section III of the book.

4. Although I will not expand on the issue here, there are clear resonances between Heidegger and Boss on bodyhood and the approach developed later by Merleau-Ponty, in his very influential *Phenomenology of Perception*. The following quotation serves to make this connection:

> The thing is inseparable from a person perceiving it, and can never be actually in itself, because its articulations are those of our very existence, and because it stands at the other end of our gaze, or at the terminus of a sensory exploration which invests it with humanity. To this extent, every perception is a communication or a communion . . . the complete expression outside ourselves of our perceptual powers, and a coition, so to speak, of our body with things.
>
> (Merleau-Ponty 1962: 320)

5. There are strong resonances between this approach to the notion of illness and that developed (from within a different philosophical tradition) by Fulford in his *Moral Theory and Medical Practice* (1989).

6. Binswanger himself called this a 'productive misunderstanding'!

Chapter 7

1. This conclusion has also emerged from an empirical, anthropological literature that has been alluded to above in Chapter 4.
2. Like many other terms used by Heidegger there has been dispute about the proper translation of the German word *Angst* into English. The translators of *Being and Time* use the word anxiety and this appears to be used by most commentators. However the word 'dread' is also used commonly. This is the word commonly used to translate *Angst* in the work of Kierkegaard.
3. In the world of medicine a great deal of knowledge about human physiology has been developed through an understanding of disease.
4. There is an older tradition within psychology which foregrounds questions of meaning. This is centred on the work of Victor Frankl. He was a native Austrian who was himself a survivor of the Nazi concentration camps. In his book *Man's Search for Meaning* (1959) he outlined his concept of logotherapy. This became the name for a school of psychotherapy that was based on helping people come to terms with the central existential questions of life's meaning and purpose. Magomed-Eminov (1997) writes that Frankl's ideas had a substantial influence on the approach to PTSD developed in the former Soviet countries in recent years.
5. I propose to use the term 'post-traumatic anxiety' as being similar to Janoff-Bulman's 'disillusionment', and to distinguish this from post-traumatic fear in relation to an outside threat.
6. Dreyfus (1991: 39) notes this tension. He says: 'Heidegger seems to imply (at the end of Division I) that his fundamental ontology in *Being and Time* will be a *full clarification* of the understanding of being, and even a *science of being as such*. This idea conflicts with the presuppositions of hermeneutics.'

Chapter 8

1. In spite of this I have pointed to the fact that he returned to this focus in the *Zollikon Seminars* that took place well into the 'later period': see Chapter 6 above.
2. We noted in Chapter 6 his criticism of Binswanger on this issue. The 'Letter on Humanism' was actually written in response to certain questions posed to Heidegger by Jean Beaufort about Sartre's essay *'L'existentialism est un Humanisme'*.
3. In spite of this, as we noted in previous chapters, Heidegger's own project in *Being and Time* is an effort to get beyond our ordinary culture and language and generate an account of human reality in its universal essence.
4. However, as argued in the last chapter, I want to retain an understanding of the ontological dimension of trauma, but as a *particular* problematic of certain cultures.
5. The translators of this lecture series use the term 'attunement' for Heidegger's word *Stimmung*. This is usually translated by the word 'mood'. Our moods are perhaps the most familiar ways in which we are 'attuned' or in a 'state-of-mind'. As I understand Heidegger a *Stimmung* is one important element of the concept of *Befindlichkeit*, but the latter term also involves a further element, what John Haugeland describes as 'the fluid involved rapport of a craftsperson or athlete with

the current work or play situation, and even the attentive responsiveness that is
prerequisite to "disinterested" observation' (Haugeland 2000: 52).

Heidegger stresses that attunement should not be regarded as a 'side effect' of
some other phenomenon. Indeed, attunement itself is the fundamental basis upon
which Dasein can begin to have any experience at all:

> Attunements are the fundamental ways in which we *find* ourselves
> *disposed* in such and such a way. Attunements are the '*how*' [*Wie*]
> according to which one is in such and such a way. Certainly we often
> take this 'one in such and such a way' . . . as something indifferent, in
> contrast to *what* we intend to do, *what* we are occupied with, or *what*
> will happen to us. And yet this 'one is in such and such a way' is not – is
> never – simply a consequence or side-effect of our thinking, doing,
> acting. It is – to put it crudely – the presupposition for such things, the
> 'medium' within which they first happen.
>
> (Heidegger 1995: 67–68)

6. Dreyfus points to the essay 'The way back into the ground of metaphysics', and I
   quote from this below.
7. Hypertrophy is a medical term that refers to an increase in the size of an organ or
   tissue due to an increase in the size of its constituent specialized cells. Physiological
   forms of hypertrophy occur in skeletal muscle due to hard work and in the muscle
   of the uterus (the myometrium) due to pregnancy. In pathological forms of hypertrophy the organ or tissue is affected by a disease process. While it is enlarged, it is
   also rendered weak. This happens in some forms of muscular dystrophy.

Chapter 9

1. I will not enter the debate about whether the term 'late modernity' would be a
   more accurate description of our current times (this term is used by Anthony
   Giddens). This does not have direct relevance to the argument to be developed
   here, as we shall see below.
2. Jean-Francois Lyotard's book *La Condition Postmoderne* was published in 1979,
   the year before PTSD was established in *DSM III*.
3. Another example is the way in which our distress has been brought into the
   domain of selling and consumption through the rise of the pharmaceutical industry and the medicalization of sadness and anxiety. For an excellent account of the
   marketing of tranquillizers and anti-depressants, see Healy (1997) *The Antidepressant Era*. See also Breggin (1983) *Psychiatric Drugs: Hazards to the Brain*, and
   Johnstone (2000) *Users and Abusers of Psychiatry*.

Chapter 10

1. The relationship between social change and suicide is complex. Famously,
   Durkheim (1951) made a link between a loss of social coherence, order and meaning and suicide. He coined the term 'anomic suicide'. However, on a global level,
   suicide is probably related more to social factors such as poverty, unemployment

and domestic violence. There is no definite relationship between technological development and suicide. For unexplained reasons, Sri Lanka has the highest suicide rate in the world. For an excellent discussion of global trends, see the chapter on suicide in Desjarlais et al. (1995) *World Mental Health: Problems and Priorities in Low-income Countries*.

2. In this book I have focused mainly on insights generated through philosophy and in particular the sort of phenomenology developed by Heidegger. My sociological and anthropological references are 'strategic' rather than comprehensive. For an excellent sociological account of mental health and its practitioners, see Pilgrim and Rogers (1999), *A Sociology of Mental Health and Illness*.

3. A good example is the fact that large companies now have departments of 'human resources', people who are available to the company, to be used in different ways.

4. This was also seen in the writing of Boss: see Chapter 7.

5. Lyotard famously wrote: 'I define postmodern as incredulity toward metanarratives' (Lyotard 1992: 138).

6. This is explored in a number of the later works and is the central concern of the essays in Heidegger (1971) *On the Way to Language*.

Chapter 11

1. This report was the result of a two-year collaborative project involving many authorities on mental health from around the world and produced through the Department of Social Medicine at Harvard University.

2. In fact the development of psychiatric nosology is not as neutral or objective as many of the scientists involved would have us believe. For an interesting discussion of how a great deal of psychiatric classification has been shaped by the marketing dynamics of the pharmaceutical industry, see Healy (1997) *The Antidepressant Era*.

3. I agree with Fred Newman and Lois Holzman (1997) that when Marx is understood primarily as an advocate of 'revolutionary *activity*' there is no contradiction between Marxism and the insights of postmodernism. In this regard, his most important observation was that 'the philosophers have only *interpreted* the world, in various ways; the point is to *change* it' (Marx 1977: 123).

4. There is now a 'user literature' on mental health. A good introduction is the collection of articles in Read and Reynolds (1996), *Speaking Our Minds: An Anthology*. See also Campbell (1993).

5. For various perspectives on hearing voices see Romme and Escher (1993), *Accepting Voices*.

References

Ager A (1997) Tensions in the psychosocial discourse: implications for the planning of interventions with war-affected populations. Development in Practice 7: 402–7.

APA (1952) Diagnostic and Statistical Manual of Mental Disorders, (1st edn). Washington, DC: American Psychiatric Association.

APA (1968) Diagnostic and Statistical Manual of Mental Disorders, (2nd edn). Washington, DC: American Psychiatric Association.

APA (1980) Diagnostic and Statistical Manual of Mental Disorders, (3rd edn). Washington, DC: American Psychiatric Association.

APA (1987) Diagnostic and Statistical Manual of Mental Disorders, (3rd edn, revised). Washington, DC: American Psychiatric Association.

APA (1994) Diagnostic and Statistical Manual of Mental Disorders, (4th edn). Washington, DC: American Psychiatric Association.

Austin JL (1980) How to Do Things with Words, (2nd edn). Oxford: Oxford University Press.

Bauman Z (1989) Modernity and the Holocaust. Oxford: Polity Press.

Bauman Z (1991) Modernity and Ambivalence. Cambridge: Polity Press.

Bauman Z (1993) Postmodern Ethics. Oxford: Blackwell.

Beaumont PJV (1992) Phenomenology and the history of psychiatry. Australian and New Zealand Journal of Psychiatry 26: 532–45.

Beck AT (1972) The Diagnosis and Management of Depression. Philadelphia: University of Pennsylvania Press.

Beck AT (1976) Cognitive Therapy and Emotional Disorders. New York: Meridan–New American Library.

Beck U (1992) Risk Society: Towards a New Modernity. London: Sage.

Becker JV, Skinner LJ, Abel GG, Axelrod R, Cichon J (1984) Sexual problems of sexual assault survivors. Women and Health 9: 5–20.

Berger P, Berger B, Kellner H (1974) The Homeless Mind. Harmondsworth: Penguin Books.

Bernstein RJ (1983) Beyond Objectivism and Relativism: Science, Hermeneutics and Praxis. Oxford: Basil Blackwell.

Bernstein RJ (ed.) (1985) Habermas and Modernity. Cambridge: Polity Press.

Blake DD, Albano AM, Keane TM (1992) Twenty years of trauma: psychological abstracts 1970 through 1989. Journal of Traumatic Stress 5; 477–84.

Bolton D, Hill J (1996) Mind, Meaning and Mental Disorder: The Nature of Causal

Explanation in Psychology and Psychiatry. Oxford: Oxford University Press.

Boss M (1958) The Analysis of Dreams. (trans. AJ Pomerans) New York: Philosophical Library.

Boss M (1963) Psychoanalysis and Daseinanalysis. (trans. L Lefebre) New York: Basic Books.

Boss M (1977) I Dreamt Last Night . . . (trans. S Conway) New York: Gardner Press.

Boss M (1979) Existential Foundations of Medicine and Psychology. (trans. S Conway, A Cleaves) New York: Jason Aronson.

Boss M (1988a) Martin Heidegger's Zollikon Seminars. (trans. B Kenny) In Hoeller K (ed.), Heidegger and Psychology. Seattle: Review of Existential Psychology and Psychiatry.

Boss M (1988b) Recent consideration in daseinanalysis. Humanistic Psychologist 16: 58–74.

Bracken P (1993) Post-empiricism and psychiatry: meaning and methodology in cross-cultural research. Social Science and Medicine 36: 265–72.

Bracken P (1994) Psychological Responses to War and Violence in Africa: A Report from Uganda. Cork: National University of Ireland, MD Thesis.

Bracken P (1995) Beyond liberation: Michel Foucault and the notion of a critical psychiatry. Philosophy, Psychiatry and Psychology 2: 1–13.

Bracken P (1999) Phenomenology and psychiatry. Current Opinion in Psychiatry 12: 593–96.

Bracken P (2001) Postpsychiatry in action: the radical possibilities of Home Treatment. In Brimblecombe N (ed.), Acute Mental Health Care in the Community: Intensive Home Treatment. London: Whurr Publishers.

Bracken P, Petty C (eds) (1998) Rethinking the Trauma of War. London: Free Association Press.

Bracken P, Thomas P (2001) Postpsychiatry: a new direction for mental health. British Medical Journal 322: 724–27.

Bracken P, Giller J, Summerfield D (1995) Psychological responses to war and atrocity: the limitations of current concepts. Social Science and Medicine 40: 1073–82.

Breggin P (1983) Psychiatric Drugs: Hazards to the Brain. New York: Springer.

Breuer J, Freud S (1955) Studies on Hysteria. Standard Edition, Vol. 2. London: Hogarth Press.

Brewin C (1996) Foreword. In Bolton D, Hill J (eds), Mind, Meaning and Mental Disorder: The Nature of Causal Explanation in Psychology and Psychiatry. Oxford: Oxford University Press.

Brown GS, Harris T (1978) The Social Origins of Depression: A Study of Psychiatric Disorder in Women. New York: The Free Press.

Button G, Coulter J, Lee J, Sharrock W (1995) Computers, Minds and Conduct. Cambridge: Polity Press.

Cambridge Dictionary of Philosophy (1995) General editor: Audi R. Cambridge: Cambridge University Press.

Campbell P (1993) Mental health services: the user's view. British Medical Journal 306: 848–50.

Campbell P (1996) What we want from crisis services. In Read J, Reynolds J (eds), Speaking Our Minds: An Anthology. Basingstoke: Macmillan Press/Open University.

Caputo JD (1993) Heidegger and theology. In Guignon C (ed.), The Cambridge Companion to Heidegger. Cambridge: Cambridge University Press.

Cilliers P (1998) Complexity and Postmodernism: Understanding Complex Systems. London: Routledge.

Collins J (2000) Heidegger and the Nazis. Cambridge: Icon Books.

Condrau G (1988) A seminar on daseinanalytic psychotherapy. Humanistic Psychologist 16: 101–29.

Connolly WE (1993) Beyond good and evil: the ethical sensibility of Michel Foucault. Political Theory 21: 365–89.

Craig E (1988a) Daseinanalysis: a quest for essentials. Humanistic Psychologist 16: 1–23.

Craig E (1988b) Freud's Irma dream: a daseinanalytic reading. Humanistic Psychologist 16: 203–16.

Crane T (1995) The Mechanical Mind. London: Penguin.

Csordas TJ (1994) Introduction: the body as representation and being-in-the-world. In Csordas TJ (ed.), Embodiment and Experience: The Existential Ground of Culture and the Self. Cambridge: Cambridge University Press.

Curran PS (1988) Psychiatric aspects of terrorist violence: Northern Ireland 1969–1987. British Journal of Psychiatry 153: 470–75.

Dallmayr F (1991) Life-World, Modernity and Critique: Paths between Heidegger and the Frankfurt School. Cambridge: Polity Press.

Daly R (1983) Samuel Pepys and post-traumatic stress disorder. British Journal of Psychiatry 143: 64–68.

de Beistegui M (1998) Heidegger and the Political: Dystopias. London: Routledge.

Deleuze G, Guattari F (1977) Anti-Oedipus: Capitalism and Schizophrenia. New York: Athlone Press.

Derrida J (1988) Limited Inc. Evanston, IL: Northwestern University Press.

Descartes R (1968) Discourse on Method and the Meditations. (ed. FE Sutcliffe) London: Penguin Books.

Desjarlais R, Eisenberg L, Good B, Kleinman A (1995) World Mental Health: Problems and Priorities in Low-Income Countries. New York: Oxford University Press.

Dreyfus H (1991) Being-in-the-World: A Commentary on Heidegger's Being and Time. Cambridge: MIT Press.

Dreyfus H (1993) Heidegger on the connection between nihilism, art, technology, and politics. In Guignon C (ed.), The Cambridge Companion to Heidegger. Cambridge: Cambridge University Press.

Dreyfus H (1994) What Computers Still Can't Do: A Critique of Artificial Reason. Cambridge: MIT Press.

Dreyfus H (2000) Responses. In Wrathall M, Malpas J (eds), Heidegger, Authenticity, and Modernity: Essays in Honour of Hubert L. Dreyfus, Vol. 1. Cambridge, MA: The MIT Press.

Durkheim E (1951) Suicide. (trans. JA Spaulding, G Simpson) Glencoe: Illinois Free Press (Macmillan).

Eisenbruch M (1991) From post-traumatic stress disorder to cultural bereavement: diagnosis of Southeast Asian refugees. Social Science and Medicine 33: 673–80.

Epstein S (1991) The self-concept, the traumatic neurosis, and the structure of personality. In Ozer D, Healy JM, Stewart AJ (eds), Perspectives on Personality, Vol. 3. London: Jessica Kingsley.

Farrell K (1998) Post-traumatic Culture: Injury and Interpretation in the Nineties. Baltimore: The John Hopkins University Press.

Faulconer JE, Williams RN (1985) Temporality in human action: an alternative to positivism and historicism. American Psychologist 40: 1179–88.

Feenberg A (1999) Questioning Technology. London: Routledge.

Fell JP (1992) The familiar and the strange: on the limits of praxis in the early Heidegger. In Dreyfus HL, Hall H (eds), Heidegger: A Critical Reader. Oxford: Blackwell.

Fenichel O (1946) The Psychoanalytic Study of Neurosis. London: Routledge and Kegan Paul.

Foa E, Steketee G, Rothbaum B (1989) Behavioral/cognitive conceptualizations of post-traumatic stress disorder. Behavior Therapy 20: 155–76.

Fodor J (1995) The persistence of attitudes. In Lyons W (ed.), Modern Philosophy of Mind. London: Everyman.

Fogelson RM (1970) Violence and grievances: reflections on the 1960s riots. Journal of Social Issues 26: 141–63.

Follesdal D (2000) Absorbed coping: Husserl and Heidegger. In Wrathall M, Malpas J (eds), Heidegger, Authenticity, and Modernity: Essays in Honour of Hubert L. Dreyfus, Vol. 1. Cambridge, MA: The MIT Press.

Foucault M (1971) Madness and Civilization: A History of Insanity in the Age of Reason. London: Tavistock.

Foucault M (1977a) Discipline and Punish. (trans. A Sheridan) London: Allen Lane.

Foucault M (1977b) Revolutionary action: 'Until now'. In Bouchard D (ed.), Michel Foucault: Language, Counter-Memory, Practice. Oxford: Blackwell.

Foucault M (1980) Michel Foucault: Power/Knowledge, Selected Interviews and Other Writings 1972–1977. (ed. C Gordon) Hemel Hempstead, England: Harvester.

Foucault M (1981) The History of Sexuality, Vol. 1. London: Penguin.

Foucault M (1983) On the genealogy of ethics. In Dreyfus H, Rabinow P (eds), Michel Foucault: Beyond Structuralism and Hermeneutics, (2nd edn). Chicago: University of Chicago Press.

Foucault M (1984) Politics and ethics: an interview. In Rabinow P (ed.), The Foucault Reader. New York: Pantheon Books.

Foxen P (2000) Cacophony of voices: a K'iche' Mayan narrative of remembrance and forgetting. Transcultural Psychiatry 37: 355–81.

Frank E, Stewart BD (1984) Depressive symptoms in rape victims. Journal of Affective Disorders 1: 269–77.

Frankl V (1959) Man's Search for Meaning. New York: Washington Square Press/Pocket Books.

Fraser N (1981) Foucault on modern power: empirical insights and normative ambiguities. Praxis International 1: 272–87.

Friedman MJ, Marsella AJ (1996) Posttraumatic stress disorder: an overview of the concept. In Marsella AJ, Friedman MJ, Gerrity ET, Scurfield RM (eds), Ethnocultural Aspects of Posttraumatic Stress Disorder: Issues, Research, and Clinical Applications. Washington: American Psychological Association.

Freud S (1920) Beyond the Pleasure Principle. Standard Edition, Vol. 18. London: Hogarth Press. pp 1–68.

Fulford KWM (1989) Moral Theory and Medical Practice. Cambridge: Cambridge University Press.

Fulford KWM (1994) Closet logics: hidden conceptual elements in the DSM and ICD classifications of mental disorders. In Sadler JZ, Wiggins OP, Schwartz MA (eds),

Philosophical Perspectives on Psychiatric Diagnostic Classification. Baltimore: The John Hopkins University Press.

Furedi F (1997) Culture of Fear: Risk-Taking and the Morality of Low Expectation. London: Cassell.

Gaines AD (1992a) Ethnopsychiatry: The Cultural Construction of Professional and Folk Psychiatries. Albany: State University of New York Press.

Gaines AD (1992b) From DSM-I to III-R; voices of self, mastery and the other: a cultural constructivist reading of U.S. psychiatric classification. Social Science and Medicine 35: 3–24.

Geertz C (1973) The Interpretation of Cultures. New York: Basic Books.

Gendlin ET (1988) Befindlichkeit: Heidegger and the philosophy of psychology. In Hoeller K (ed.), Heidegger and Psychology. Seattle: Review of Existential Psychology and Psychiatry.

German GA (1987) The nature of mental disorder in Africa today II: some clinical observations. British Journal of Psychiatry 151: 440–46.

Gergen K (1995) Metaphor and monophony in the 20th-century psychology of emotions. History of the Human Sciences 8(2): 1–23.

Giddens A (1991) Modernity and Self-Identity: Self and Society in the Late Modern Age. Cambridge: Polity Press.

Giller JE (1998) Caring for 'victims of torture' in Uganda: some personal reflections. In Bracken P, Petty C (eds), Rethinking the Trauma of War. London: Free Association Books.

Giller JE, Bracken PJ, Kabaganda S (1991) Uganda: war, women and rape. Lancet 337: 604.

Goffman E (1971) Relations in Public: Micro Studies of the Public Order. New York: Basic Books.

Goldstein K (1939) The Organism: A Holistic Approach to Biology. New York: The American Book Company.

Goleman D (1985) Vital Lies, Simple Truths: The Psychology of Self-deception. New York: Simon and Schuster.

Good BJ, Good MD (1982) Towards a meaning-centred analysis of popular illness categories: 'fright-illness' and 'heart-distress' in Iran. In Marsella AJ, White GM (eds), Cultural Conceptions of Mental Health and Therapy. Dordrecht: D. Reidel.

Gordon C (1990) Histoire de la Folie: an unknown book by Michel Foucault. History of the Human Sciences 3: 3–26.

Gordon DR (1988) Tenacious assumptions in Western medicine. In Lock M, Gordon DR (eds), Biomedicine Examined. Dordrecht: Kluwer Academic Publishers.

Greenley JR, Gillespie DP, Lindenthal JJ (1975) A race riot's effects on psychological symptoms. Archives of General Psychiatry 32: 1189–95.

Grinker K, Spiegal S (1945) Men under Stress. Philadelphia: Blakeston.

Haar M (1992) Attunement and thinking. In Dreyfus H, Hall H (eds), Heidegger: A Critical Reader. Oxford: Blackwell.

Habermas J (1987) The Philosophical Discourse of Modernity. Cambridge: Polity Press.

Hacking I (1995) Rewriting the Soul: Multiple Personality and the Sciences of Memory. Princeton: Princeton University Press.

Hall H (1993) Intentionality and world: Division I of Being and Time. In Guignon C (ed.), The Cambridge Companion to Heidegger. Cambridge: Cambridge University Press.

Hampson N (1968) The Enlightenment: An Evaluation of its Assumptions, Attitudes and Values. London: Penguin.

Harré R, Gillett G (1994) The Discursive Mind. Thousand Oaks: Sage Publications

Harré R, Secord PF (1973) The Explanation of Social Behaviour. Oxford: Blackwell.

Haugeland J (2000) Truth and finitude: Heidegger's transcendental existentialism. In Wrathall M, Malpas J (eds), Heidegger, Authenticity, and Modernity: Essays in Honour of Hubert L. Dreyfus, Vol. 1. Cambridge, MA: The MIT Press.

Harvey D (1989) The Condition of Postmodernity: An Enquiry into the Origins of Cultural Change. Oxford: Blackwell.

Healy D (1997) The Antidepressant Era. Cambridge, MA: Harvard University Press.

Heidegger M (1956) The way back into the ground of metaphysics. In Kaufmann W (ed.), Existentialism from Dostoevsky to Sartre. Cleveland: Meridian Books.

Heidegger M (1962) Being and Time. (trans. J Macquarrie, E Robinson) Oxford: Blackwell.

Heidegger M (1966) Discourse on Thinking. (trans. JM Anderson, EH Freund) New York: Harper and Row.

Heidegger M (1971) On the Way to Language. (trans. PD Hertz) New York: Harper and Row.

Heidegger M (1977) The Question Concerning Technology and Other Essays. (ed. W Lovitt) New York: Harper Torchbooks.

Heidegger M (1982) Nietzsche, Vol. IV: Nihilism. (trans. FA Capuzzi) New York: Harper and Row.

Heidegger M (1988) On adequate understanding of Daseinanalysis. (trans. M Eldred; notes by E Craig, P Kastrinidis). Humanistic Psychologist 16: 75–100.

Heidegger M (1993) Basic Writings. (ed. DF Krell) London: Routledge and Kegan Paul.

Heidegger M (1995) The Fundamental Concepts of Metaphysics: World, Finitude, Solitude. (trans. W McNeill, N Walker) Bloomington: Indiana University Press.

Heidegger M (2001) Zollikow Seminars. Protocols, Conversations, Letters. Edited by Boss M (trans F Mayr, R Askay) Illinois: Northwestern University Press.

Hempill RE (1941) The influence of the war on mental disease: a psychiatric study. Journal of Mental Science 87: 170–82.

Henningsen P, Kirmayer L (2000) Mind beyond the net: implications of cognitive neuroscience for cultural psychiatry. Transcultural Psychiatry 37: 467–94.

Herman J (1992) Trauma and Recovery: The Aftermath of Violence – from Domestic Violence to Political Terror. New York: Basic Books.

Hesse M (1980) Revolutions and Reconstructions in the Philosophy of Science. Bloomington: Indiana University Press.

Higginbotham N, Marsella A (1988) International consultation and the homogenization of psychiatry in Southeast Asia. Social Science and Medicine 27: 553–61.

Hobart M (1985) Anthropos through the looking-glass: or how to teach the Balinese to bark. In Overing J (ed.), Reason and Morality. London: Tavistock Publications.

Hodgkinson PE, Stewart M (1991) Coping with Catastrophe: A Handbook of Disaster Management. London: Routledge.

Hoeller K (1988) Phenomenology, psychology, and science. In Hoeller K (ed.), Heidegger and Psychology. Seattle: Review of Existential Psychology and Psychiatry.

Horgan J (1999) The Undiscovered Mind: How the Brain Defies Explanation. London: Weidenfeld and Nicolson.

Horowitz MJ (1986) Stress Response Syndromes. New Jersey: Jason Aronson.

Horowitz MJ, Willner N, Alvarez W (1979) Impact of events scale: a study of subjective stress. Psychosomatic Medicine 41(3): 209–18.

Hume D (1962) A Treatise on Human Nature, Book One. (ed. DGC Macnabb) Glasgow: Fontana/Collins. (Originally published in 1739).

Ingleby D (1980) Critical Psychiatry. New York: Pantheon Books.

Jameson F (1991) Postmodernism, or the Cultural Logic of Late Capitalism. London: Verso.

Janoff-Bulman R (1992) Shattered Assumptions: Towards a New Psychology of Trauma. New York: The Free Press.

Jaspers K (1963) General Psychopathology. (trans. J Hoenig, MW Hamilton) Manchester: Manchester University Press.

Jenkins J (1991) The state construction of affect: political ethos and mental health among Salvadorean refugees. Culture, Medicine and Psychiatry 15: 139–65.

Jenkins J (1996) Culture, emotion, and PTSD. In Marsella AJ, Friedman MJ, Gerrity ET, Scurfield RM (eds), Ethnocultural Aspects of Posttraumatic Stress Disorder. Washington, DC: American Psychological Association.

Jenkins JH, Karno M (1992) The meaning of expressed emotion: theoretical issues raised by cross-cultural research. American Journal of Psychiatry 149: 9–21.

Johnstone L (2000) Users and Abusers of Psychiatry, (2nd edn). London: Routledge.

Joseph S, Williams R, Yule W (1997) Understanding Post-traumatic Stress Disorder: A Psychosocial Perspective on PTSD and Treatment. Chichester: John Wiley and Sons.

Kant I (1992) What is Enlightenment. In Eliot S, Whitlock K (eds), The Enlightenment: Texts II. Milton Keynes: The Open University.

Keane TM, Zimmerling RT, Caddell JM (1985) A behavioral formulation of post-traumatic stress disorder in Vietnam veterans. The Behavior Therapist 8: 9–12.

Kelly GA (1955) The Psychology of Personal Constructs. New York: Norton.

Kiev A (1972) Transcultural Psychiatry. Harmondsworth: Penguin.

Kilpatrick DG, Veronen LJ, Best CL (1985) Factors predicting psychological distress among rape victims. In Figley CR (ed.), Trauma and its Wake, Vol. 1. New York: Brunner/Mazel.

Kirmayer L (1996) Confusion of the senses: implications of ethnocultural variations in somatoform and dissociative disorders for PTSD. In Marsella AJ, Friedman MJ, Gerrity ET, Scurfield RM (eds), Ethnocultural Aspects of Posttraumatic Stress Disorder: Issues, Research, and Clinical Applications. Washington: American Psychological Association.

Kleinman A (1977) Depression, somatization and the 'New cross-cultural psychiatry'. Social Science and Medicine 11: 3–10.

Kleinman A (1980) Patients and Healers in the Context of Culture. Berkeley: University of California Press.

Kleinman A (1987) Anthropology and psychiatry: the role of culture in cross-cultural research on illness. British Journal of Psychiatry 151: 447–54.

Kleinman A (1988) Rethinking Psychiatry: From Cultural Category to Personal Experience. New York: The Free Press.

Kleinman A, Good B (1985) Culture and Depression. Berkeley: University of California Press.

Kovel J (1988) The Radical Spirit: Essays on Psychoanalysis and Society. London: Free Association Press.

Krystal JH, Kosten TR, Perry BD, Southwick SM, Mason JW, Giller EL (1989) Neurobiological aspects of PTSD: review of clinical and preclinical studies. Behavior Therapy 20: 177–98.

Kulka RA, Schlenger WE, Fairbank JA, Hough RL, Jordan BK, Marmar CR, Weiss DS (1990) Trauma and the Vietnam War Generation: Report of Findings from the National Vietnam Veterans Readjustment Study. New York: Brunner/Mazel.

Kutchins H, Kirk S (1999) Making Us Crazy. DSM: The Psychiatric Bible and the Creation of Mental Disorders. London: Constable.

Laing RD (1967) The Politics of Experience and The Bird of Paradise. Harmondsworth: Penguin.

Lash S (1990) Sociology of Postmodernism. London: Routledge.

Lee D, Turner S (1997) Cognitive-behavioural models of PTSD. In Black D, Newman M, Harris-Hendriks J, Mezey G (eds), Psychological Trauma. London: Gaskell.

Leff J (1988) Psychiatry Around the Globe. London: Royal College of Psychiatrists.

Leff J (1990) The 'New cross-cultural psychiatry': a case of the baby and the bathwater. British Journal of Psychiatry 156: 305–7.

Levin DM (1987) Psychopathology in the epoch of nihilism. In Levin DM (ed.), Pathologies of the Modern Self: Postmodern Studies on Narcissism, Schizophrenia, and Depression. New York: New York University Press.

Levin JD (1992) Theories of the Self. Washington: Hemisphere Publishing Corporation.

Levinas E (1978) Existence and Existents. (trans. A Lingus) The Hague: Martinus Nijhoff.

Lifton RJ (1967) Death in Life: Survivors of Hiroshima. New York: Simon and Schuster.

Lifton RJ (1988) Understanding the traumatized self: imagery, symbolization, and transformation. In Wilson JP (ed.), Human Adaptation to Extreme Stress. New York: Plenum.

Lindy J (1996) Psychoanalytic psychotherapy of posttraumatic stress disorder: the nature of the therapeutic relationship. In van der Kolk BA, McFarlane AC, Weisaeth L (eds), Traumatic Stress: The Effects of Overwhelming Experience on Mind, Body, and Society. New York: The Guilford Press.

Littlewood R (1990) From categories to contexts: a decade of the 'new cross-cultural psychiatry'. British Journal of Psychiatry 156: 308–27.

Littlewood R, Lipsedge M (1986) The 'culture-bound syndromes' of the dominant culture: culture, psychopathology and biomedicine. In Cox J (ed.), Transcultural Psychiatry. London: Croom Helm.

Lloyd D (1994) Connectionist hysteria: reducing a Freudian case study to a network model. Philosophy, Psychiatry and Psychology 1: 69–88.

Lock M (1982) Popular conceptions of mental health in Japan. In Marsella AJ, White GM (eds), Cultural Conceptions of Mental Health and Therapy. Dordrecht: Reidel.

Lyons HA (1972) Depressive illness and aggression in Belfast. British Medical Journal 1: 342–45.

Lyons W (1995) Introduction. In Lyons W (ed.), Modern Philosophy of Mind. London: Everyman.

Lyotard JF (1984) The Postmodern Condition: A Report on Knowledge. Manchester: Manchester University Press.

Lyotard JF (1992) Answering the question: what is postmodernism? In Jencks C (ed.), The Post-Modern Reader. London: Academy Editions.

McCall RJ (1983) Phenomenological Psychology: An Introduction. Madison: University of Wisconsin Press.

McCann IL, Pearlman LA (1990) Psychological Trauma and the Adult Survivor: Theory, Therapy, and Transformation. New York: Brunner/Mazel.

McCulloch G (1995) The Mind and its World. London: Routledge.

McFarlane A (1989) The aetiology of post-traumatic morbidity: predisposing, precipitating and perpetuating factors. British Journal of Psychiatry 154: 221–28.

McLellan D (1977) Karl Marx: Selected Writings. Oxford: Oxford University Press.

Magomed-Eminov MS (1997) Post-traumatic stress disorders as a loss of the meaning of life. In Halpern DF, Voiskounsky AE (eds), States of Mind: American and Post-Soviet Perspectives on Contemporary Issues in Psychology. Oxford: Oxford University Press.

Manes C (1992) Nature and silence. Environmental Ethics 14: 339–50.

Marmar CR, Weiss DS, Pynoos RS (1995) Dynamic psychotherapy of post-traumatic stress disorder. In Friedman MJ, Charney DS, Deutch AY (eds), Neurobiological and Clinical Consequences of Stress: From Normal Adaptation to PTSD. Philadelphia: Lippincott-Raven Publishers.

Marsella AJ (1982) Culture and mental health: an overview. In Marsella AJ, White GM (eds), Cultural Conceptions of Mental Health and Therapy. Dordrecht: Reidel.

Marsella AJ, Friedman MJ, Gerrity ET, Scurfield RM (1996a) Preface. In Marsella AJ, Friedman MJ, Gerrity ET, Scurfield RM (eds), Ethnocultural Aspects of Posttraumatic Stress Disorder: Issues, Research, and Clinical Applications. Washington, DC: American Psychological Association.

Marsella AJ, Friedman MJ, Spain EH (1996b) Ethnocultural aspects of PTSD: an overview of issues and research directions. In Marsella AJ, Friedman MJ, Gerrity ET, Scurfield RM (eds), Ethnocultural Aspects of Posttraumatic Stress Disorder: Issues, Research, and Clinical Applications. Washington DC: American Psychological Association.

Marx K (1977) Theses on Feuerbach. In Marx K, Engels F (ed. CJ Arthur), The German Ideology. London: Lawrence and Wishart.

May R (1977) The Meaning of Anxiety, (revd. edn). New York: WW Norton and Co.

Mayer-Gross W, Slater E, Roth M (1960) Clinical Psychiatry. London: Cassell.

Meichenbaum D (1997) Treating Post-Traumatic Stress Disorder: A Handbook and Practice Manual for Therapy. Chichester: John Wiley and Sons.

Merleau-Ponty M (1962) Phenomenology of Perception. London: Routledge and Kegan Paul.

Mill JS (1953) A System of Logic – Selections. In Weiner PP (ed.), Readings in Philosophy of Science. New York: Scribner's.

Mira E (1939) Psychiatric experience in the Spanish Civil War. British Medical Journal 1: 1217–20.

Mollica R, Wyshak G, Lavelle J (1987) The psychosocial impact of war trauma and torture on Southeast Asian refugees. American Journal of Psychiatry 144: 1567–72.

Mott FW (1919) War Neuroses and Shell Shock. London: Oxford Medical Publications.

Mowrer OH (1960) Learning Theory and Behavior. New York: Wiley.

Mulhall S (1996) Heidegger and Being and Time. (Routledge Philosophy Guidebook Series) London: Routledge.

Newell A, Simon HA (1963) GPS: a program that simulates human thought. In Feigenbaum EA, Feldman J (eds), Computers and Thought. New York: McGraw-Hill.

Newman F, Holzman L (1997) The End of Knowing: A New Developmental Way of Learning. London: Routledge.

Obeyesekere G (1985) Depression, Buddhism, and the work of culture in Sri Lanka. In Kleinman A, Good B (eds), Culture and Depression: Studies in the Anthropology and Cross-Cultural Psychiatry of Affect and Disorder. Berkeley: University of California Press.

O'Brien LS (1994) What will be the psychiatric consequences of the war in Bosnia? British Journal of Psychiatry 164: 443–47.

O'Brien S (1998) Traumatic Events and Mental Health. Cambridge: Cambridge University Press.

O'Brien T (1990) How to tell a true war story. In O'Brien T, The Things They Carried. Boston: Houghton Mifflin.

Olafson F (1987) Heidegger and the Philosophy of Mind. New Haven: Yale University Press.

Orbach S (1986) Hunger Strike: The Anorectic's Struggle as a Metaphor for our Age. London: Faber and Faber.

Parker I (1998) Against postmodernism: psychology in cultural context. Theory and Psychology 8(5): 601–27.

Phillips J (1996) Hermeneutics. Philosophy, Psychiatry, and Psychology 3: 61–69.

Pilgrim D, Rogers A (1999) A Sociology of Mental Health and Illness, (2nd edn). Buckingham: Open University Press.

Polkinghorne D (1984) Methodology for the Human Sciences. Albany: State University of New York Press.

Polt R (1999) Heidegger: An Introduction. London: UCL Press.

Porter R (1987) A Social History of Madness: Stories of the Insane. London: Weidenfeld and Nicolson.

Porter R (1997) The Greatest Benefit to Mankind: A Medical History of Humanity from Antiquity to the Present. London: Harper Collins.

Putnam H (1962) What theories are not. In Nagel E, Suppes P, Tarsky A (eds), Logic, Methodology, and the Philosophy of Science: Proceedings of the 1960 International Congress. Stanford: Stanford University Press.

Putnam H (1975) Mind, Language and Reality, Philosophical Papers, Vol. 2. Cambridge: Cambridge University Press.

Putnam H (1988) Representation and Reality. Cambridge, MA: MIT Press.

Read J, Reynolds J (eds) (1996) Speaking Our Minds: An Anthology. Basingstoke: Macmillan Press/Open University.

Richardson W (1963) Heidegger: Through Phenomenology to Thought. The Hague: Nijhoff.

Richardson W (1993) Heidegger among the doctors. In Sallis J (ed.) Reading Heidegger: Commemorations. Bloomington: Indiana University Press.

Ritterman M (1987) Torture: the counter-therapy of the state. Networker, Jan/Feb: 43–47.

Romme M, Escher S (1993) Accepting Voices. London: Mind Publications.

Rorty R (1979) Philosophy and the Mirror of Nature. Princeton: Princeton University Press.

Rorty R (1980) A reply to Dreyfus and Taylor. Review of Metaphysics 34: 41.

Rose N (1989) Governing the Soul. London: Routledge.

Roth M, Kroll J (1986) The Reality of Mental Illness. Cambridge: Cambridge University Press.

Rothbaum BO, Foa EB (1996) Cognitive-behavioral therapy for posttraumatic stress disorder. In van der Kolk BA, McFarlane AC, Weisaeth L (eds), Traumatic Stress: The Effects of Overwhelming Experience on Mind, Body, and Society. New York: The Guilford Press.

Rouse J (1987) Knowledge and Power: Towards a Political Philosophy of Science. New York: Cornell University Press.

Sainsbury Centre for Mental Health (1998) Acute Problems: A Survey of the Quality of care in Acute Psychiatric Wards. London: The Sainsbury Centre.

Safranski R (1998) Martin Heidegger: Between Good and Evil. (trans. E Osers) Cambridge, MA: Harvard University Press.

Samson C (1995) The fracturing of medical dominance in British psychiatry? Sociology of Health and Illness 17: 245–68.

Sass L (1989) Humanism, hermeneutics, and humanistic psychoanalysis: differing conceptions of subjectivity. Psychoanalysis and Contemporary Theory 12: 433–504.

Sass L (1990) The truth-taking stare: a Heideggerian interpretation of a schizophrenic world. Journal of Phenomenological Psychology 21(2): 121–49.

Sass L (1992a) Heidegger, schizophrenia and the ontological difference. Philosophical Psychology 5(2): 109–32.

Sass L (1992b) Madness and Modernism: Insanity in the Light of Modern Art, Literature and Thought. Cambridge: Harvard University Press.

Schank RC, Abelson RP (1977) Scripts, plans and knowledge. In Johnson-Laird PN, Wason PC (eds), Thinking: Readings in Cognitive Science. New York: Cambridge University Press.

Schepple KL, Bart PB (1983) Through women's eyes: defining danger in the wake of sexual assault. Journal of Social Issues 39: 63–81.

Scott CE (1975) Daseinanalysis: an interpretation. Philosophy Today 19: 182–97.

Scott W (1990) PTSD in DSM III: a case in the politics of diagnosis and disease. Social Problems 37: 294–310.

Sedgwick P (1982) Psychopolitics. New York: Harper and Row.

Shephard B (2000) A War of Nerves: Soldiers and Psychiatrists 1914–1994. London: Jonathan Cape.

Sheridan A (1980) Michel Foucault: The Will to Truth. London: Tavistock Publications.

Shore JH, Vollmer WM, Tatum EL (1989) Community patterns of posttraumatic stress disorder. Journal of Nervous and Mental Disease 177: 681–85.

Shweder RA, Bourne EJ (1982) Does the concept of the person vary cross-culturally? In Marsella AJ, White GM (eds), Cultural Conceptions of Mental Health and Therapy. Dordrecht: Reidel.

Skolbekken J (1993) The risk epidemic in medical journals. Social Science and Medicine 40: 296.

Slife BD (1993) Time and Psychological Explanation. Albany: State University of New York Press.

Smart B (1993) Postmodernity. London: Routledge.

Smith Q (1981) On Heidegger's theory of moods. The Modern Schoolman 58: 211–35.

Solomon RC (1988) Continental Philosophy since 1750: The Rise and Fall of the Self. Oxford: Oxford University Press.

Steiner G (1978) Heidegger. Glasgow: Fontana.

Summerfield D (1991) The rise of post-traumatic stress disorders. British Medical Journal 303: 1271.

Summerfield D (1996) The Impact of War and Atrocity on Civilian Populations: Basic Principles for NGO Interventions and a Critique of Psychosocial Trauma Projects. London: Relief and Rehabilitation Network, ODI.

Summerfield D (1997) The impact of war and atrocity on civilian populations. In Black D, Newman M, Harris-Hendriks J, Mezey G (eds), Psychological Trauma: A Developmental Approach. London: Gaskell.

Summerfield D (1998) The social experience of war and some issues for the humanitarian field. In Bracken P, Petty C (eds), Rethinking the Trauma of War. London: Free Association Press.

Summerfield D, Toser L (1991) 'Low intensity' war and mental trauma in Nicaragua: a study in a rural community. Medicine and War 7: 84–99.

Taylor C (1980) Understanding in human science. Review of Metaphysics 34: 25–38.

Taylor C (1989) Sources of the Self: The Making of the Modern Identity. Cambridge: Harvard University Press.

Taylor C (1993) Engaged agency and background in Heidegger. In Guignon C (ed.), The Cambridge Companion to Heidegger. Cambridge: Cambridge University Press.

Tillich P (1952) The Courage To Be. New Haven: Yale University Press.

Titchener J (1986) Post-traumatic decline: a consequence of unresolved destructive drives. In Figley CR (ed.), Trauma and its Wake, Vol. 2. New York: Brunner/Mazel.

van der Kolk BA (1996) The body keeps the score: approaches to the psychobiology of posttraumatic stress disorder. In van der Kolk BA, McFarlane AC, Weisaeth L (eds), Traumatic Stress: The Effects of Overwhelming Experience on Mind, Body, and Society. New York: The Guilford Press.

van der Kolk BA, McFarlane AC (1996) The black hole of trauma. In van der Kolk BA, McFarlane AC, Weisaeth L (eds), Traumatic Stress: The Effects of Overwhelming Experience on Mind, Body, and Society. New York: The Guilford Press.

van Velsen C (1997) Psychoanalytical models. In Black D, Newman M, Harris-Hendriks J, Mezey G (eds), Psychological Trauma: A Developmental Approach. London: Gaskell.

Wakefield J (1988) Hermeneutics and empiricism: commentary on Donald Meichenbaum. In Messer S, Sass L, Woolfolk R (eds), Hermeneutics and Psychological Theory. New Brunswick, New Jersey: Rutgers University Press.

Welte B (1982) The question of God in the thought of Heidegger. Philosophy Today 26: 85–100.

White GM, Marsella AJ (1982) Introduction. In Marsella AJ, White GM (eds), Cultural Conceptions of Mental Health and Therapy. Dordrecht: Reidel.

White SK (1991) Political Theory and Postmodernism. Cambridge: Cambridge University Press.

Wittgenstein L (1980) Remarks on the Philosophy of Psychology, Vol. 2. (ed. GH von Wright, H Nyman) Chicago: University of Chicago Press.

Wrathall M, Malpas J (2000) Heidegger, Authenticity, and Modernity: Essays in Honour of Hubert L. Dreyfus, Vol. 1. Cambridge, MA: The MIT Press.

Yehuda R, Giller EL, Levengood RA, Southwick SM, Siever LJ (1995) Hypothalamic-pituitary-adrenal functioning in post-traumatic stress disorder: expanding the concept of the stress response spectrum. In Friedman MJ, Charney DS, Deutch AY (eds), Neurobiological and Clinical Consequences of Stress: From Normal Adaptation to PTSD. Philadelphia: Lippincott-Raven Publishers.

Yehuda R, McFarlane A (1995) Conflict between current knowledge about posttraumatic stress disorder and its original conceptual basis. American Journal of Psychiatry 152: 1705–13.

Young A (1995) The Harmony of Illusions: Inventing Post-Traumatic Stress Disorder. Princeton: Princeton University Press.

Zarowsky C (2000) Trauma stories: violence, emotion and politics in Somali Ethiopia. Transcultural Psychiatry 37: 383–402.

Zarowsky C, Pedersen D (2000) Rethinking trauma in a transnational world. Transcultural Psychiatry 37: 291–93.

Zimmerman ME (1993) Heidegger, Buddhism, and deep ecology. In Guignon C (ed.), The Cambridge Companion to Heidegger. Cambridge: Cambridge University Press.

Index

Abelson, R. P., 36
acute stress disorder, 48–49
adaptation process, 210
Adorno, T., 186
Ager, Alastair, 211
agoraphobia, 183
alienation, 164, 173–175, 179
American Civil War, 66
American Psychiatric Association, 31
anorexia nervosa, 183–184
anti-psychiatry, 223
anxiety, 133–138
    and death, 2–3, 138–140, 172
    modernity and meaning, 170–173
    rethinking the place of, 151–156
Aristotle, 27, 106, 158, 229n.6
artificial intelligence (AI)
    background knowledge, 145–146
    cognitivism, 38–39
    Heidegger, 100–101
    meaning and intelligibility, 93, 94
asylums, 19–20
Austin, J. L., 198, 199
authenticity, 164
    anxiety, rethinking the place of,
        151–156
    Heidegger's later works, 156–157
    history of being and critique of
        modernity, 157–159
    subjectivity and modernity,
        162–164
    technology and nihilism, 159–162
Axis V scale, 74

Balinese culture, 102–103
Bart, P. B., 54
Bauman, Zygmunt, 176, 196–197, 202,
    203
Beaufort, Jean, 233n.2
Beck, Aaron, 36–37
Beck, Ulrich, 181
Becker, J. V., 50
Befindlichkeit, 131–133
behaviourism
    Heidegger's philosophy contrasted
        with, 121
    limitations, 38
    post-traumatic stress disorder, 49–51
being, history of, 157–159
being-in-the-world, 87–88
    anxiety, 152, 153–154
    structure, 130–131
    Zollikon seminars, 113
        Binswanger, 121
        'bodyhood' and illness, 114, 115
Berger, P., 181
Bernstein, R. J., 231n.2
Binswanger, Ludwig, 120–121
biomedicine, 28
Blake, D. D., 45
Bleuler, Eugen, 112, 120, 184
bodyhood, see embodiment
Bolton, Derek, 10–11
    cognitivism, 25–26, 101–102, 103
    functionality in biological science, 105
    meaning, 144
    positivism, 33
    post-traumatic stress disorder, 56

boredom, 155
Bosnia, 217
Boss, Medard, 11, 86, 112–113
    'bodyhood' and illness, 113–116, 143
    daseinanalysis, 122
        dream interpretation, 123–124
        limitations, 127–128
        and psychoanalysis, 122–123
        therapeutic attitude, 126–127
    on Freud, 117–119
    stress, 121–122
Bourne, E. J., 212–213
Bowlby, John, 58
Breuer, Josef, 51
Brewin, Chris, 10
Brown, G. S., 103, 230n.10
Buddhism, 195
Button, G., 26, 43

calculative thinking, 191
Cambodian refugees, 71–72, 74
Campbell, Peter, 227
capitalism, 173–175, 179
Caputo, John, 194–195
care, 120–121, 134–135
Cartesianism, 8, 21
    cogito, 21
        Heidegger's reversal of, 90–92
    and cognitivism, 25–27, 39
    as 'common sense' of Western culture,
        11
    dualism, 22–23
    Husserl's phenomenology and
        modern psychiatry, 24–25
    limitations, 110–111
    reason and certainty, 21–22
causality, 75–77
    cognitivism, 41–42
    Heidegger's philosophy, 101–105, 149
        temporality, 107
    positivism, 31, 76
    post-traumatic stress disorder, 61–62,
        77–80
certainty, Cartesian understanding of,
    21–22
Chomsky, Noam, 36
Cilliers, Paul, 44
civil indifference, 147

classical learning, 49–50
cognitivism, 10–11, 33–37
    and Cartesianism, 25–27
    emergence, 37–39
    functionalism, 39–41
    Heidegger's philosophy, 101–102
    and hermeneutics, difference
        between, 141
    limitations, 63–65, 80–81
        historical aspects, 65–67
        linear causality, 75–80
        social context, 67–75
    'magic circle', 57, 59–60
    philosophical assumptions, 39–41
    popularity, increasing, 33–34
    post-traumatic stress disorder, 53–54
        cognitive appraisal, 54–55
        information-processing, 55–56
    time and causality, 41–42
    trauma, meaning and science, 60–61,
        148
collective trauma, 70
Collins, Jeff, 87
completion tendency, 53, 55–56
computer model, 38–40, 53–54
    see also artificial intelligence (AI)
Comte, Auguste, 27
Condrau, Gion, 123, 124
connectionism, 43–44
Connolly, W. E., 200
consumerism, 14, 179–180
conversion hysteria, 66
cortisol abnormalities, 79–80
countertransference, 53
Craig, Erik, 124–125, 126, 127
cross-cultural psychiatry, 212–220
    'old' and 'new', 214–220
    relevance, 212–214
Csordas, Thomas, 230n.1
cultural bereavement, 71–72
cultural context, 210–211
    emotion, 72–75
    Heidegger's philosophy, 86
        meaning and intelligibility, 95
        scientific reductionism and
            positivism, 104–105
    social distancing, 146
    war and violence, 71–72
    see also cross-cultural psychiatry

culture-bound syndromes, 182–183
Curran, P. S., 69

Dallmayr, F., 117
Daly, R., 65
Dasein
    anxiety, 134–138, 140, 152, 153–154,
        155
    and death, 139
    attunements, 234n.5
    Cartesian cogito, reversal of, 90, 91
    change in Heidegger's philosophy,
        151–152, 156, 157
    concept, 88–90
    meaning
        and intelligibility, 92
        ontological approach, 144, 147,
            149
    mood
        Befindlichkeit, 132
        structure of being-in, 130, 131
    scientific reductionism and positivism,
        99–100
    temporality, 105–106, 107,
        108–109, 110
    Zollikon seminars, 113
        'bodyhood' and illness, 114, 115
        critique of Binswanger, 120–121
daseinanalysis, 120, 122
    dream interpretation in, 123–124
    limitations, 127–128
    and psychoanalysis, 122–123
    therapist's 'attitude', 124–127
death, and anxiety, 2–3, 138–140, 172
death imprint, 142
de Beistegui, Miguel, 193–194
deductive-nomological system, 29–30
deep ecology, 195
Deleuze, G., 185
depression
    causality, 103–104
    cognitive therapy, 36–37
    postmodernity, 186
    war, 68–69
Derrida, Jacques, 198, 199
Descartes, René
    metaphysics, 162–163
    reason, 19

subjectivism, 186
    see also Cartesianism
Desjarlais, R., 210–211
developmental psychology, 35
Diagnostic and Statistical Manual, 221
    positivism, 31
    post-traumatic stress disorder, 45–46,
        47, 61–62
    linear causality, 77, 79
    syndrome, 47–49
Dilthey, Wilhelm, 98–99, 153, 154,
    231n.2
disillusionment, 141–142
disordered action of the heart, 66
dissociation, 73
distance-standing, 146
distress, postmodern, 182–187
dreams, 75
    daseinanalysis, 123–125, 126
Dreyfus, Hubert, 12, 13
    Cartesianism, 21, 23, 26
    Heidegger, 12, 13, 231n.2
        anxiety, 137, 155
        artificial intelligence, 145–146
        Befindlichkeit, 132
        Christian narrative, 155
        Dasein, 89, 231n.4
        hermeneutics, 233n.1
        meaning and intelligibility, 93–94
        scientific reductionism and
            positivism, 98–101
        sense, 147
        social distancing, 146
        social world, 153, 154
        technology, 159, 192
    Husserl, 229n.4
Durkheim, Emile, 67, 69, 234n.1

Eisenbruch, Maurice, 71–72
eliminative materialism, 39
embodiment, 86
    meaning and intelligibility, 92–94, 145
    scientific reductionism and positivism,
        98
    Zollikon seminars, 113–116
Emergency PsychoSocial Care, 217
emotion and culture, 72–75

empiricism, 27, 28–29, 38, 229n.5
Enframing, 160–161, 191, 193–194, 214, 218
Enlightenment, European, 17–21
    Cartesianism, 21–27
    science and positivism, 27–33
        causality, 31, 75–76
epistemology, 17
Erikson, Eric, 58
ethical issues
    postpsychiatry, 224–225
    'responsibility for otherness', 196–197, 199–202
existentialism in Heidegger's philosophy, 151–152, 154–155
expressed emotion, cultural context, 104
externalist accounts of mind, 26, 43

false memory, 7
Farrell, Kirby, 2–3
Faulconer, J. E., 107
fear
    culture of, 181–182
    Heidegger's philosophy, 133–134, 135–136, 140, 171
Feenberg, Andrew, 222
Fell, Joseph, 138
feminism, 63–64
Feyerabend, Paul K., 98
First World War, 66
Foa, E. B., 51, 54
Fodor, Jerry, 39, 40–41
Follesdal, Dagfinn, 229n.4
Foucault, Michel, 162
    ethical sensibility, 199–201, 214
    Kantian revolution, 186
    psychiatry, 19, 20, 32–33
Foxen, Patricia, 7–8
Frank, E., 54
Frankl, Victor, 233n.4
Fraser, N., 201
Freud, Sigmund
    Boss, 113, 123, 127
    completion tendency, 55
    dream interpretation, 123, 124–125, 126
    Heidegger on, 116–120
    hysteria, 51–52

influence, 225–226
post-traumatic stress disorder, 64
repetition compulsion, 53
Friedman, M. J., 230n.1
Fulford, K. W. M., 4–5, 227, 232n.5
functionalism, 39–41
Furedi, Frank, 181–182

Gadamer, Hans-Georg, 13
Gelassenheit, 191–194, 199, 207, 214, 218
    drawing a positive agenda from, 194–196
Gendlin, E. T., 132, 133
Gergen, Kenneth, 38
German, G. A., 215
Gestalt psychology, 94
Gestell (Enframing), 160–161, 191, 193–194, 214, 218
Giddens, A., 177–178, 180
    anorexia nervosa, 184
    late modernity, 234n.1
    ontological security, 147
Giller, Joan, 208, 219
Gillett, Frant, 34, 35, 105
Goffman, Erving, 147, 202
Goldstein, Kurt, 136
Goleman, Daniel, 36
Gordon, Deborah, 28
Great Fire of London, 65
Grinker, K., 66
Guatemala, 7, 148
Guattari, F., 185

Habermas, J., 193, 198–199, 221
Hacking, Ian, 6–7
Hall, Harrison, 97–98
Hampson, Norman, 17–18
Harré, Rom, 34, 35, 36, 105
Harris, T., 103, 230n.10
Harvey, D., 224
Haugeland, John, 233–234n.5
Hearing Voices Network, 227
Heidegger, Martin, 8–9, 11–13, 85–86, 110–112, 128–129
    anxiety, 151–156, 170–171, 172, 173, 206–207

Boss and the Zollikon seminars,
112–113
Binswanger, 120–121
'bodyhood' and illness, 113–116
Freud, Heidegger on, 116–120
stress, 121–122
change in philosophy, 151
controversy, 12, 86–87
daseinanalysis, 88–90, 122
dream interpretation in, 123–124
limitations, 127–128
and psychoanalysis, 122–123
therapist's 'attitude', 124–127
Gelassenheit, 191–196, 207, 214, 218
hermeneutic phenomenology, 206
individualism and 'internal' accounts
of mind, 87–96
being-in-the-world, 87–88
Cartesian cogito, reversal of, 90–91
dasein concept, 88–90
meaning and intelligibility, 91–96
Janoff-Bulman's 'new psychology of
trauma', 141–142, 143
later works, 156–157
history of being and modernity
critique, 157–159
subjectivity and modernity,
162–164
technology and nihilism, 159–162,
186, 221
meaning, ontological approach,
143–145, 147
mood
Befindlichkeit, 131–133
being-in, structure of, 130–131
postmodernity, move to, 176
post-traumatic stress disorder, 79
scientific reductionism and positivism,
96–110
intentional causality, 101–105
significance, 96–101
temporality and historicality,
105–110
helplessness, learned, 103
Hempill, R. E., 68
Herman, Judith, 63–64, 168
hermeneutics
and cognitivism, difference between,
141

Heidegger, 13, 99–100, 152, 154–155
phenomenology, 206
Hesse, Mary, 27, 98
Higginbotham, N., 215–216
Hill, Jonathan, 10–11
cognitivism, 25–26, 101–102, 103
functionality in biological science, 105
meaning, 144
positivism, 33
post-traumatic stress disorder, 56
Hobart, M., 102–103
Hodgkinson, P. E., 209
Hoeller, Keith, 228n.3
Holzman, Lois, 235n.3
Horgan, John, 101
Horney, Karen, 113
Horowitz, Mardi, 59, 60, 62, 77
completion tendency, 53, 55–56
normal stress response, exaggeration
of, 79
humanism, 152, 163
human rights, 7–8
Hume, David, 29
Husserl, Edmund, 86
Cartesian cogito, 231–232n.5
Heidegger's reorientation of
phenomenology, 13
phenomenology, Cartesian
orientation of, 24–25
hypothalamic-pituitary-adrenal (HPA)
axis, 79–80
hysteria, 51, 66

illness, 115–116, 143
Impact of Events Scale, 74
individualism, Heidegger's critique
being-in-the-world, 87–88
Cartesian cogito, reversal, 90–91
Dasein, 88–90
meaning and intelligibility, 91–96
information-processing models, 35
Heidegger's philosophy, 94, 95
post-traumatic stress disorder, 55–56
Ingleby, David, 31, 223
instrumental learning, 49–50
intellectuals, specific, 201
intelligibility, Heidegger on, 91–96
irritable heart, 66

Jameson, F., 224
Janoff-Bulman, Ronnie
    'new psychology of trauma', 56–60,
        140–143
    schemas, 36
Jaspers, Karl, 24–25, 225
Jenkins, Janis, 70, 72, 104
Joseph, S., 210
Jung, Carl, 113, 120, 124

Kabaganda, Stella, 219
Kant, Immanuel, 18, 186, 231–2n.5
Karno, Marvin, 104
Kierkegaard, S., 153, 154, 155, 161,
        233n.2
Kiev, A., 215
Kilpatrick, D. G., 50
Kirk, S., 221
Kirmayer, Laurence, 73–74
Kleinman, Arthur, 167–168, 212, 214,
        226
Kohli-Kunz, 118–119
Koro, 183
Kovel, J., 223
Kraepelin, Emil, 184
Kroll, Jerome, 32
Kuhn, Thomas, 98
Kutchins, H., 221

Laing, R. D., 185, 223
language, 198–199
Lash, Scott, 177
learned helplessness, 103
learning theory, 49–51
Lee, D., 61
Leff, J., 215
Levin, David, 186
Levin, Jerome, 19
Levinas, Emmanuel, 231n.4
Lewis, Aubrey, 25
libido theory, 117
Lifton, Robert, 142
Lindy, Jacob, 53
Lipsedge, M., 182–183
Littlewood, Roland, 182–183, 215
Lloyd, Dan, 230n.12
Lock, Margaret, 212
logotherapy, 233n.4

London, Great Fire of, 65
Lovitt, W., 160
Luther, Martin, 170
Lyons, H. A., 68–69
Lyotard, Jean-Francois, 197, 234n.2,
        235n.5

McCall, R. J., 89, 132, 231n.4
McCulloch, G., 26, 43
McFarlane, A. C., 9, 62, 78–79, 205
Macquarrie, J., 89, 125, 131–132
madness, postmodern, 182–187
magic circle of everyday life, 1–5, 56–60,
        64–65
Magomed-Eminov, M. S., 233n.4
Manes, Christopher, 195
Marmar, C. R., 52, 53
Marsella, A. J., 212, 215–216, 218–219,
        230n.1
Marx, Karl
    alienation, 164, 173–175, 179
    postmodernism, 235n.3
materialism, eliminative, 39
May, Rollo, 173, 180
Mayan Indians, 7, 148
Mayer-Gross, W., 30
meaning, 1–4
    approaches to, 8–9
        phenomenological, 11–13
        postmodern, 13–14
        psychiatric, 9–11
    cognitivism, 56–57, 64–65
    Heidegger on, 91–96
    modernity, 168–173, 206–207
        Marx and the question of
        alienation, 173–175
    ontological exploration, 143–150
    philosophy and politics of, 5–8
    postmodernity, decline of 'meaning'
        within, 176–179, 206–207
    psychiatric approach to loss of,
        208–212
meaninglessness, postmodern response,
        220–223
medical model of psychiatry, 30–31
meditative thinking, 191
memory
    active, 55–56

cognitivism, 42, 76–77
false, 7
philosophy and politics of, 5–8
post-traumatic stress disorder, 55–56, 77
temporality, 109–110
Merleau-Ponty, M., 232n.4
metaphysics, 137, 156–157, 158, 162
Mill, John Stuart, 27
Mira, Emilio, 68
modernity
Heidegger's philosophy, 155–156, 157–159, 162–164
meaning, question of, 168–173, 206–207
Marx and the question of alienation, 173–175
mood, Heidegger's understanding of
Befindlichkeit, 131–133
being-in, structure of, 130–131
moral beliefs, 169–171
Mount St Helens volcano eruption, 78
Mowrer, O. H., 49
Mulhall, Stephen, 144
multiple personality disorder, 7
music, meaning of, 94–95

Nagel, Thomas, 92
narcissism, 186
naturalism, 28–29
nature, 96–97, 98–100
Nazism, Heidegger, 86–87, 112, 196
Negi Negi, 183
neurasthenia, 66
Newell, A., 39
Newman, Fred, 235n.3
Newtonian physics, 76
Nicaragua, 74
Nietzsche, Friedrich, 87, 161, 162, 186
nightmares, 75
nihilism, 159–162, 186
non-governmental organizations (NGOs), 213, 217–218, 220
Northern Ireland, 68–69

Obeyesekere, Gannanath, 103–104
O'Brien, S., 65–66
O'Brien, Tim, 142

Olafson, Frederick, 23
Heidegger's engagement with
Descartes, 162–163
memory, 42, 109–110
technology, 161
temporality, 106, 108, 109–110
ontic inquiry, 13
ontological inquiry, 13
meaning, 143–150
Orbach, Susie, 184
organic movement, 222
otherness, 'responsibility for', 196–202

parapraxis, 117–118
Parker, I., 224
Pedersen, D., 219
Pepys, Samuel, 65
Personal Construct Theory, 35–36
personality theory, 35
phenomenology
Heidegger
'bodyhood', 116
critique of Freud, 117
meaning, 144–150
hermeneutic, 206
Husserl's, 24–25
meaning, 9–11, 228n.4
Phillips, J., 228n.5
philosophy of meaning and memory, 5–8
phobias, 49, 51
Piaget, Jean, 35
Plato, 106, 158
politics of meaning and memory, 5–8
Polkinghorne, D., 27–28
Polt, Richard, 110–111, 164
Porter, Roy, 19, 20, 224–225
positivism, 26–33
causality, 31, 76
cognitivism, 34–35, 64–65
Heidegger's critique, 96–110
postmodernity
madness and distress, 182–187
meaning
approach to, 13–14
decline of, 176–179, 206–207
meaninglessness, responding to, 220–223
move to, 175–182

decline of 'meaning' within
  postmodernity, 176–179
postpsychiatry, 224
responding to, 189–191, 202–203
  Gelassenheit, 191–196
  'responsibility for otherness',
    196–202
subjectivity, 179–182
postpsychiatry, 223–227
  contextualist understanding and
    practice, 225–226
  ethical issues, foregrounding, 224–225
  power differentials, recognition of,
    226–227
post-traumatic stress disorder (PTSD),
  45–47, 62
  behavioural approaches, 49–51
  cognitivism, 53–54
    cognitive appraisal, 54–55
    information-processing, 55–56
  creation of diagnosis, 46–47, 67
  cross-cultural psychiatry, 217,
    218–219
  current discourse, 205
  Diagnostic and Statistical Manual,
    45–46, 47, 61–62
  linear causality, 77, 79
  syndrome, 47–49
  diagnostic framework, 9
  Herman, 64
  Janoff-Bulman's 'new psychology of
    trauma', 56–60
  limitations of cognitivism
    historical aspects, 65–67
    linear causality, 75–80
    social context, 67, 70, 73–74, 75
  meaning and science, 60–62
  positivism, 65
  postmodernity, 182, 187
  psychodynamic contributions, 51–53
  syndrome, 47–49
  trauma, meaning and science, 61
processing of trauma, 208–209
Protagoras, 158
psychiatry
  approach to meaning, 11–13, 208–12
  Cartesian orientation, 24–25
  cross-cultural

'old' and 'new', 214–220
  relevance, 212–214
diagnosis, problems with, 4
Enlightenment, 18–20
positivism, 30–33
psychoanalysis, 122–123
psychodynamic theory, 51–53
psychology
  Enlightenment, 18–20
  Husserl's phenomenology, 24
psychopathology, 30
psychopharmacology, 221
psychotherapy, relevance of, 212–214
Putnam, Hilary
  computer functionalism, 39–40
  externalist accounts of mind, 43
  'received view', 28

rape victims, 50, 54, 69
rationalism, 27, 229n.5
  anthropology, 102–103
  cognitivism, 38
Rayner, 49
reason
  Cartesian understanding of, 21–22
  Enlightenment, 17–18, 19, 20
reductionism, 96–110
reflection, 90–91
refugees, cultural bereavement, 71–72
religion
  anxiety, 170
  commodification, 14
  decline in Western cultures, 6–7
  orderliness of the world, 58
  variety, 75
  see also spiritualism
repetition compulsion, 53
repression, 117–119
'responsibility for otherness', 196–202
Ricoeur, Paul, 13
riots, 68–69
Robinson, E., 89, 125, 131–132
Rorty, Richard, 228n.5
Rosaldo, 72
Rose, Nikolas, 179–180
Roth, Sir Martin, 30, 32
Rothbaum, B. O., 51
Rouse, Joseph, 99–100, 162

Rwanda, 217
Ryle, Gilbert, 43

Safranski, Rüdiger, 86, 87, 228n.2,
    232n.1
Sainsbury Centre, 202
Sartre, Jean-Paul, 152, 201, 233n.2
Sass, Louis, 10, 24, 90, 187, 228
    schizophrenia, 184, 185–186
Schank, R. C., 36
schemes, 53
    cognitivism, 36–37, 54, 56
    Janoff-Bulman, 58
Schepple, K. L., 54
schizophrenia, 184–186
science
    Heidegger's critique, 96–110
    postmodernity, 178
    and psychiatry, 27–30
        positivism, 30–33
    trauma and meaning, 60–62
Scott, Charles, 89
Scott, Wilbur, 46, 47
Searle, John, 198
Second World War, 66–68
Sedgwick, Peter, 32
seduction theory, 51–52
self, Enlightenment, 18–19
Seligman, 103
shell shock, 66
Shephard, Ben, 66, 209
Sheridan, Alan, 33
Shweder, R. A., 212–213
significance, 96–101, 116
Simon, H. A., 39
Skolbekken, J., 181
Slater, E., 30
Slife, Brent, 76, 94
Smart, B., 14
social distancing, 146
social world, 60
    culture and emotion, 72–75
    Heidegger, 153–154
    Janoff-Bulman, 60
    war and violence, 67–72
sociocentric cultures, 212–213
soldier's heart, 66
solicitude, 125–127

Solomon, Robert, 18
somatization, 67, 73
Spanish Civil War, 68
speech-act theory, Austin, 198
Spengler, Oswald, 87
Spiegal, S., 66
spiritualism
    anxiety, 172–173
    decline in Western cultures, 7
    orderliness in the world, 58
    variety, 75
    see also religion
Sri Lanka, 235n.1
Steiner, George, 11–12, 87, 91
    meaning and intelligibility, 95
Stewart, B. D., 54
Stewart, M., 209
stress, 121–122
subjectivity
    Heidegger, 162–164
    postmodern, 179–182
Sudanese civil war, 70–71
suicide, 190
Summerfield, Derek, 70–71, 74, 148,
    217–218

Taylor, Charles, 92–93
    modernity and meaning, 168–171
    scientific reductionism and positivism,
        98–99, 100
technology, 221–222
    Heidegger, 159–162, 163–164
        Boss, 128–129
        Gelassenheit, 192, 193–194, 196
Thomas, Phil, 222–223
Tillich, Paul, 171–173
time
    cognitivist framework, 41–42, 75–77
        post-traumatic stress disorder,
        61–62, 77–80
    Heidegger's approach, 105–110, 149
Titchener, James, 52
torture, 69–70
Toser, L., 74
transcendence, 229n.3
transcendental standpoint, Husserl, 24
transference, 53
trust, 58

truth commissions, 6
Tuke family, 224–225
Turing machine functionalism, 40
Turner, S., 61

Uganda, 5–6, 74, 208, 219–220
United Nations (UN), 213, 220
universalism, psychological, 35
user movement, 227

van der Kolk, B. A., 9, 49
Van Velsen, C., 53
Veterans Administration (VA), 46
Vienna Circle, 29
Vietnam War
    opposition to, 64
    post-traumatic stress disorder, 46–47,
        50, 77, 209
violence, 67–72
von Gebsattel, 232n.1

Wakefield, Jerome, 41
war, 67–72, 74
    see also specific wars
Watson, 49
Welte, Bernard, 195
White, G. M., 212

White, Stephen, 197–198, 199, 203
Williams, R. N., 107
Wittgenstein, Ludwig
    being-in-the-world, 154
    change in philosophy, 151
    externalist accounts of mind, 43
    meaning, 144, 145
    rule-following psychological activity,
        105
worldliness, 96–97, 98
World War I, 66
World War II, 66–68

Yehuda, R., 62, 78, 79–80
Young, Allan
    post-traumatic stress disorder
        causality, 80
        creation, 46–47, 67, 168, 205
        intrusion-avoidance symptoms,
            78–79
        temporality, 61
    stress, 122

Zarowsky, Christina, 213, 219
Zen Buddhism, 195
Zimmerman, Michael E., 156, 195

9 781861 562807